1994

Cost Management Strategies
for Smaller Hospitals

Malcolm R. Hastings
for the Section for Small or Rural Hospitals
of the American Hospital Association

American Hospital Publishing, Inc., an American Hospital Association company

Library of Congress Cataloging-in-Publication Data

Hastings, Malcolm R.
    Cost management strategies for smaller hospitals / Malcolm R. Hastings.
        p.   cm.
    Includes bibliographical references
    ISBN 1-55648-105-5 (pbk.)
    1. Hospitals—Cost Control   I. Title
    [DNLM: 1. Cost Control—methods. 2. Financial Management, Hospital. 3. Economics, Hospital—United States. WX 157 H358c 1993]
    RA971.3.H265   1993
    362.1'1'0681—dc20
    DNLM/DLC
    for Library of Congress   93-1908
                                            CIP

Catalog no. 184131

©1993 by American Hospital Publishing, Inc.,
an American Hospital Association company

Printed in the USA

𝔸ℍ𝔸 is a service mark of the American Hospital Association used under license by American Hospital Publishing, Inc.

CCN, Inc. and San Diego Community Healthcare Alliance use the name Community Care Network as their service mark and reserve all rights.

Text set in Palacio
2.5M—07/93—0349

Richard Hill, Acquisitions and Development Editor
Lee Benaka, Production Editor
Peggy DuMais, Production Coordinator
Luke Smith, Cover Designer
Marcia Bottoms, Books Division Assistant Director
Brian Schenk, Books Division Director

To Kathy, Patrick, and Jeanne for their love. To Peggy Wolf for teaching and working with me. To Fred Gould for giving me a start in health care. To the people at Hyatt, Imler, Ott & Blount, whose creative genius helps many hospitals complete their mission.

Contents

List of Figures and Tables

About the Author

Malcolm R. Hastings is principal in charge of health care consulting for Hyatt, Imler, Ott & Blount (HIOB), a health care consulting and accounting firm in Atlanta, Georgia. His work as a consultant extends to helping several smaller hospitals to improve profitability through implementing operational improvements and other innovations. Before joining HIOB, the author was responsible for the turnaround management of a fifty-bed hospital. He has also worked with several administrators as the vice-president of operations for a multihospital system. In addition, he has served as a trustee for three small hospitals.

Mr. Hastings holds a bachelor of arts degree in economics from Washington and Lee University in Lexington, Virginia.

Foreword

Today we are in the midst of discussions about national health care reform. Though no one can predict with certainty the outcome of these discussions, it is likely that health care reform will embrace certain principles, namely, the efficient use of technology, personnel, and health care dollars; access to care for those without adequate health care coverage; a delivery system that shifts the balance toward prevention and somewhat away from intervention; approaches to health care that offer a demonstrable link between the use of health care resources and the improvement in health status of the population; and the creation of a health care system that provides accountability and assurances of quality to the payer.

Meanwhile, what can hospitals do to position themselves for the changes that are coming? How can small hospitals—which, in general terms, have fewer resources and face tougher economic and demographic challenges to their survival—be proactive *today* to minimize the trauma that is always part of any change? These are the key questions that are addressed in this book.

A critical assumption inherent in the writing of this book is that smaller hospitals are less-complex organizations than larger hospitals. Generally, smaller hospitals have fewer layers of management staff, and each manager usually handles several aspects of hospital operations. This centralized administration often makes decision making easier.

Smaller hospitals also serve well-defined communities. The hospitals are located in geographically distinct towns, and the people living in each hospital's primary service area are easily identified. A sense of community is easily fostered; when the hospital's survival is threatened, the community usually rallies to support its key economic and service institution. Those who predicted the demise of hundreds of smaller, rural hospitals between 1980 and 1990 failed to recognize the strength of this support and loyalty. Such predictions did not come to pass because the people in those communities gave dollars directly and through taxes to support their hospitals.

It must always be remembered, however, that smaller hospitals must make operational and management decisions with limited resources and capital reserves. With such narrow margins for error, it is critical for smaller and undercapitalized hospitals to make the right decisions. Decision-makers require accurate, appropriate, and timely information about current hospital operations.

The best source of this information is within the hospital. By involving members of hospital management, staff nurses, physicians, and employees of the hospital, critical information on hospital costs can be collected. This theme of collaboration leading to cost-controlling information runs throughout Mr. Hastings's book, and is a key to the survival of smaller hospitals. Obviously, this book will not be able to save all small hospitals, but for existing hospitals that enjoy community support and are required to make appropriate strategic decisions, this book promises to be very helpful.

Kim C. Byas
Senior Staff Specialist
Section for Small or Rural Hospitals
American Hospital Association
Chicago, Illinois
May 1993

Preface

Reduced inpatient utilization . . . less-favorable payer mixes . . . physician recruitment barriers . . . skilled manpower shortages. . . . Although these are challenges for all hospitals, no sector has been hit harder than the smaller hospital. Many smaller hospitals have closed, and more are in receivership or just barely making payroll each month.

At a time when innovation in health care delivery is most needed, the funds to make the transition are nonexistent for smaller hospitals. As a result, the successful smaller hospital sets an example for other providers to follow by making improvements in delivery through relatively small expenditures. The key is efficiently using available resources and appropriately responding to environmental changes.

Most hospitals were built for a time that no longer exists. Reforms in regulations and payment are changing the way hospitals do business. The age of predominant inpatient utilization and cost-based reimbursement is fading away. In the future, there will be more emphasis on diagnostics, surgery, and treatment being done on an outpatient basis, in the physician's office, and in the patient's home. Over the next 10 to 15 years, payment for services covered by most carriers will shift to a predominantly capitated basis. Inpatient care, as it is known today, will be used selectively for highly resource-consumptive cases. The smaller hospital, which has not traditionally treated resource-consumptive patients, will divert available capital expenditures to ancillary departments and convert unused inpatient areas to alternative functions such as observation, holding, and respite care beds. This trend has already been accepted by most smaller hospitals.

Hospitals were enticed to the outpatient market through the continuation of cost-based reimbursement when the prospective payment system for Medicare inpatient services was initiated in 1983. Today, outpatient services (largely physician payments) have become Medicare's fastest-growing expenditure area, and this area is beginning to undergo significant payment reform as well.

In an effort to control Medicare Part B expenditures, there have been continued changes in the payment process for most Medicare outpatient services. Hospitals have shifted from cost-based payment to the use of CPT codes and the lesser of actual charges or regional prevailing rates for all services. Medicare's physician payment reform has recently introduced a new payment structure using the Resource-Based Relative Value Scale (RBRVS) for physician services. During the 1990s, further initiatives are expected in the drive to reduce Medicare expenditures to hospitals providing outpatient services.

A new era awaits hospitals as they evolve into a more cost-conscious total health care environment. Hospitals can expect to see those who pay the health care bill (the Health Care Financing Administration, commercial carriers, employers, and patients) demand more value for their money. This demand will force hospitals not only to practice cost-effective medicine, but also to demonstrate the value of the care delivered. To accomplish these goals, providers will need to accurately report cost and outcome information and correlate the severity of patient illness to the cost of treatment.

Although every health care professional acknowledges that treating a patient appropriately takes priority over choosing the treatment that results in the highest payment, many studies show that a physician's treatment behavior and a hospital's service offerings are influenced by financial incentives. Changing payment requirements and consumer expectations will require providers to structure treatment in a different manner.

Hospitals are also entering the age of chronic disease management. This concept has been discussed for years, but only recently has anything been done to make it a health care delivery focus. Chronic disease is consistently reported as the cause of most deaths and illnesses.

Treatment of chronic disease is very resource consumptive, and chronic diseases often are not detected until their later acute stages. Some reports have shown that about half of a person's total health care expenses occur in the last six months of life. When chronic diseases are diagnosed early, the course of most chronic illnesses (such as most cancer, heart problems, diabetes, renal disorders, and so forth) can be managed through early treatment interventions, changes in life-style, and behavior modifications. Hospital costs will be reduced by appropriately addressing these illnesses when they first appear.

Chronic disease management can bring new life to an efficiently run smaller hospital. Managing chronic conditions requires improved access to care. Facilities need to be close to where patients live, free of parking problems, and able to utilize efficient scheduling of procedures to minimize wasted physician and patient time. Effective health care will require minimizing the hurdles to routine patient screening and treatment.

Smaller community hospitals are positioned to meet the requirements of this new environment, but they must be prepared to deliver a higher volume of service at lower cost than in the past. This emphasis on cost control will require management and medical staff to make a sober internal review to determine what can be done better and more efficiently. Hospital management, the medical staff, and the board of trustees must understand this mission as a joint effort to identify and implement needed change.

The purpose of this book is to help smaller hospitals position themselves for a more value-driven health care environment. Although primarily addressing issues at the board and CEO level, this book attempts to help department managers and physicians in smaller hospitals gain a better understanding of broad hospital cost-containment issues. This book should also clarify management and physician roles in helping to change the way smaller hospitals deliver health care. The focus will be to provide various techniques to empower those who work for and with smaller hospitals to contain costs and fulfill the hospital's mission.

Acknowledgments

I have widely adopted the general management philosophies of Phillip Crosby and W. Steven Brown when addressing hospital performance improvement. I extend special thanks to Melissa Toler and Sharon Graves for their input and advice on various clinical issues; Kim Byas, Senior Staff Specialist, AHA Section for Small or Rural Hospitals, for his review and input of both the outline and the manuscript; Sylvia Boeder, Director, AHA Section for Small or Rural Hospitals, for her confidence; Lisa Polk for her assistance with the manuscript; and Rick Hill for his comments and dedication to the completion of this project.

Chapter 1

The Prerequisites of Survival

"We need your help. We have a real problem." Not long ago, I was surprised to hear one of our clients begin a conversation this way. Don is the chief financial officer of a very successful 100-bed county hospital in Georgia. In the past, he had engaged us from time to time to review specific areas that usually resulted in only minor adjustments, and we had never discovered any "real problems."

He went on. "We just completed our annual audit and our bottom line is even higher than it was last year. It's up to $2.3 million." The hospital had made a very respectable $1.5 million the year before. "We need to have you tell us and our board if we are making too much money. Then give us some suggestions about what we should say to our physicians." This was neither a typical request from a small hospital client nor a typical bottom line.

The situation does illustrate the existing antiprofit attitude many people have toward hospital services. Don did not have a problem with making a profit; his concern was the reaction of others to the fact that his hospital had made a profit. The truth is that a hospital cannot survive without making a profit. Administrators can dress it up as a "future expense for equipment and programs," but they still must be able to take it to the bank. A hospital must have collectible revenues in excess of expenses.

This concept often makes hospital managers in not-for-profit hospitals uncomfortable. Just as soon as a hospital reports a profit, administrators become concerned with the responses they will receive. Physicians may want to know why the piece of equipment they requested was not purchased. Employees may want to know why they did not get bigger pay raises. Members of the community may be concerned that the hospital's rates are too high.

Interestingly, Don's hospital is one of the best-equipped hospitals of its size. In addition, its average charges per discharge, when compared by one of the local insurance carriers to other hospitals, were one-third lower than the average hospital in its peer group. The hospital was not paying the highest average salary among area hospitals, but it was not offering the lowest either.

The answer was easy. By exercising effective scrutiny of its expenditures, the hospital was acting as a responsible health care provider. Through maintaining a consistently fair profit margin, a hospital can help improve the quality of care being provided to the community and, in the process, keep health care costs down. And the answer can be made clearer by exploring the scenarios of profitable hospitals versus failing hospitals.

The Failing Hospital

Declining Community Hospital felt the same effect many hospitals felt as the Medicare prospective payment system (PPS) went into effect: fewer patients and lower inpatient payments. The hospital had built up a comfortable level of cash reserves and when the annual audit report showed a loss from operations, the board members were not very concerned. They looked to management to make adjustments.

The next year's financial report again showed a loss. Management told the board that Medicare's payment increases were unjustifiably low and that inpatient utilization was down because of increased scrutiny being placed on the physicians by the peer review organization (PRO). Operational shortfalls were recouped from existing reserves, and the board, to the administration's dismay, held back on several equipment purchases that had been planned.

The physicians became frustrated, because they had always been able to look to the hospital to provide equipment as needed. The hospital's role began to be challenged as more and more equipment requests were turned down or stalled. The physicians saw themselves as "customers" (administrators did, too!). The revenue shortfalls certainly were not their fault. A business decline began, accompanied by a cash reserve erosion, as illustrated in figure 1-1.

The administrators did not want to share financial information with the physicians. Financial information was never anything the physicians were interested in. Besides, if the medical staff knew that the hospital was losing money, they would lose confidence in the hospital's management.

At the same time, the hospital began recruitment efforts to attract specialists to the medical staff. As the hospital brought in prospects, the community hosted welcoming parties to make the physician candidates and their families feel welcome. Consistently, however, these physicians remained concerned about the hospital's lack of modern equipment, as

Figure 1-1. The Effect of Eroding Cash Reserves

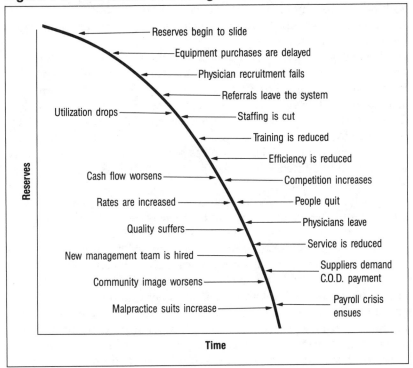

well as the hospital's poor track record for making capital expenditures over the past year.

When recruiting efforts failed, the hospital's primary care physicians were forced to send patients to specialists in a city 50 miles away. It was a longer drive for the patients, but it could usually be tied in with other errands that needed to be done in the metropolitan area.

As a result, patient loads continued to diminish because the specialists seeing the patients used hospitals close to their offices. Declining Community Hospital and its physicians even attempted to persuade the city specialists receiving the referrals to set up temporary offices in the smaller town. Although Declining Community Hospital was successful in recruiting these physicians to its community once or twice per week, hospital utilization did not increase. When patients qualified for admission, the specialist usually referred them to a larger facility in the city where "they were appropriately equipped to take care of the patient."

Despite its declining caseload, the community hospital did little to reduce staffing. Both the administration and the board felt that the hospital probably was overstaffed, but no one seemed to know in which areas or by how much. As a result, the hospital's financial problems worsened, with payroll becoming an ever-increasing drain on cash. Any hope for using cash or obtaining outside financing in the short run had become out of the question.

There was no money for training, and the supervisors did little on-the-job staff training. It was not that the supervisors did not want to train their staff; the supervisors were so busy working to make up for staff shortages that they did not have time for training. Work took less time and was done better when supervisors did it themselves anyway, or so they thought. As a result, there was no time to identify opportunities for improving efficiency. Unless subordinates took the initiative to do something differently, things just kept getting done the way they always had gotten done.

Finally, cash flow became so restricted that the hospital made two moves simultaneously. The administration froze all salaries and told department heads to reduce their staffs. Clinical departments would not be affected as much as others, but administrative departments such as medical records and the business office faced extensive cutbacks.

These moves caused three major problems. The current lack of improvement in skill level and efficiency among staff was harmful, but staff reductions made things worse. Tests were not being scheduled properly, and patients were not being prepared properly or receiving appropriate nursing care. In general, the staff reductions resulted in reduced effectiveness as well, causing physicians even more concern about the quality of nursing care being rendered.

Additionally, staff reductions in the business office and medical record department led to further cash-flow restrictions caused by longer delays in billing and collecting. With fewer personnel to make sure physicians promptly completed the inpatients' medical records (required for filing Medicare inpatient claims) and less time available to follow up on filed claims, the hospital experienced increasing payment delays.

Finally, because of the hospital's seemingly arbitrary layoffs and salary freezes, many of the most capable employees began leaving the hospital for other opportunities in a skilled labor environment where demand far exceeded supply. The loss of experienced staff only compounded the existing efficiency and quality problems.

At this point, the hospital felt that making substantial increases in rates was its only hope. Consequently, the hospital increased its charges for all services and supplies by 15 percent. Most members of the board of trustees were not excited about this idea, because many were owners of companies that employed most of the local work force. However, the administration and board could not agree on any reasonable alternative solution. As a result of price increases, the hospital's commercial patient base began to diminish.

Faced with increasing rates, little reduction in costs, restricted cash flow, low employee morale, and lower utilization rates, the hospital board decided that it was time for a change in the management team. When the new management team arrived, it quickly recognized that the only thing the hospital could do to remain in existence was to begin reducing services. The first services to be eliminated were the least profitable (obstetric and nursery services, followed by intensive care and cardiac care). Many smaller hospitals historically have chosen not to provide these services. Soon, other critical care services were reduced as well: emergency services, electrocardiograph testing, and ultrasound testing. Community members, hospital physicians, and hospital staff began wondering whether they still had a hospital.

Many hospitals have pruned unprofitable services and still remained viable health care providers. They have accomplished this by introducing alternative new services and expanding existing viable services. Along with financial investment and physician input, new service development requires the cooperation of department heads. Unfortunately, department heads at Declining Community Hospital had little time for such innovations.

Because of its restricted cash flow, the hospital was not able to pay its bills in a timely fashion. As a result, many vendors put the hospital on cost-on-delivery payment terms. Without money available to meet these terms, department heads had to become more involved in the purchasing process, calling various vendors to obtain needed supplies and services for their departments. This robbed department managers of the time needed for planning new services.

Soon the hospital was unable to make payroll. Continued operations would require a significant and continuing cash infusion if the hospital's doors were to remain open. With a deterioration of service and an inability to remain financially solvent, the hospital would be pressed to find a source of capital infusion. It was going down the financial drain.

The Successful Hospital

Progressive Community Healthcare Center has a much more positive story to tell. The hospital averages only 20 inpatients per day, but it boasts over $10 million in revenue from additional services. It has significantly expanded its outpatient service capability with an entirely new ambulatory center. The hospital features a specially designed program in industrial medicine focused on identifying health problems early and getting workers back on the job quickly. Modern cardiopulmonary testing, ultrasonography, mammography, laboratory, and radiology equipment are used constantly and replaced as necessary. Additionally, a nursing home, extended care facility, and retirement center are located on the hospital's campus. Finally, all clinical equipment and facility planning is done with the active involvement of the medical staff.

Hospital administrators present the hospital's financial position to the medical staff at their monthly meetings. As shown in figure 1-2, a constant source of cash available from operations allows the hospital to continually invest in equipment and new programs. With expanded facilities and new programs, the hospital looks more attractive to physicians. With successful recruitment and retention of physicians, the hospital can focus its attention on working with these physicians to develop new services focused on early detection and management of chronic illness.

New services mean greater career opportunities for employees. As service expansion occurs, more jobs are created. Upward movement in management also occurs as needs are identified for more talent to plan and operate the new services. The hospital is very successful in recruiting and retaining hospital employees. Employees are attracted to the hospital as a place to work because they feel that they are fulfilling their own career needs through involvement in these new services.

With plentiful resources, Progressive Community Healthcare Center provides necessary training and education to employees. The hospital maintains a continually improving environment, resulting in more efficient

Figure 1-2.   The Effect of Increasing Cash Reserves

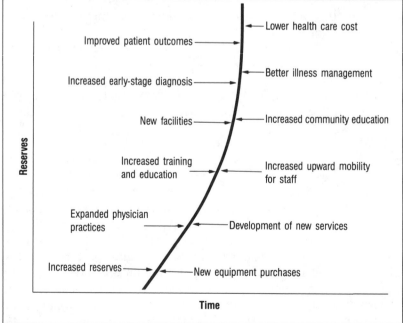

performance of duties and better patient care. Availability of continued education and training helps make the hospital a learning environment where the employees want to work and grow. Turnover is minimal.

Providing health-related information is critical to the hospital's mission to the community. The educational process focuses on making the community aware of the early warning signs of illness and the hospital's capabilities to help patients detect health problems early. This process eventually leads to timely intervention and an approach to treatment emphasizing a change in life-style. As with most of the hospital's innovations, this educational approach is possible only because funds are readily available.

Through providing continuing education and training, as well as increasing community awareness, Progressive Community Healthcare Center is improving the quality of care it offers through better patient outcomes and simultaneous reductions in health care costs. To do this, the hospital must make a profit. Making a profit means that costs must be kept in line with gradual growth. Employees are not overpaid. Staffing is monitored and compared to developed labor standards every payroll period. Department heads know that, if they are going to approach administration with a request to add staff, they had better come with facts and a plan to support the request. Budgets are well planned, adjusted, and reviewed. Any budget variances are analyzed and actions are taken on a monthly basis.

In general, Progressive Community Healthcare Center is a successful hospital. Its employees enjoy opportunities for learning and advancement, its physicians relish working with the latest equipment, and the community feels that its health care needs are being met with great skill and care. But the hospital is successful especially because its staff works hard to find ways to continuously improve.

Contributors to the Healthy Bottom Line

The activities of every individual in the hospital contribute to the bottom line. Employees directly involved in revenue centers within the hospital have at least some understanding of this fact. Everyone is involved in controlling costs. Every day there are opportunities to produce better outcomes or identify ways to accomplish the hospital's mission with less expense.

Few managers see their activities translated into instant profit or loss, but this fact should not be used as an excuse to avoid financial accountability. After a predetermined period of time, there should be an expected level of results for every hospital function.

In any business, investments are made with a time factor in mind. If an investment does not show results after a reasonable period, the course of action should be altered. Managers who dismiss their role in generating profit are often the first to see budgets for their departments trimmed as profit margins shrink. Therefore, each manager has a personal stake in contributing to the hospital's profit. This is not an obligation employees have to the chief executive officer; it is an obligation to the hospital's patients and everyone involved in delivering health care to those patients.

Managers should consider how to effectively impress upon each employee and medical staff member the link between their daily actions and the financial outcome of the hospital. Once this cause-and-effect relationship is understood by managers, employees, and medical staff, the hospital can begin building a more efficient operation. Costs can be reduced and the quality of care can improve while operating profits are maintained.

Chapter 2

Reducing Costs in the Smaller Hospital

E very hospital manager wants to contain costs. Often, however, they are not sure which costs to reduce, how far to reduce them, or how to implement the reductions. Along with pertinent, accurate data, it takes effective supervisors and workers to reduce costs. The more people involved in identifying cost savings and developing better ways to do business, the more likely it becomes that planned results will be achieved. The effective achievement of cost-containment objectives depends on the *voluntary* efforts and cooperation of everyone affected.

The Five Phases of Cost Containment

Like the maturation of an organization's quality improvement program,[1] the behavior of a hospital's management team and board goes through distinct phases as they attempt to reduce costs. In some ways, the phases of cost containment resemble the recovery process for drug or alcohol dependency.

Phase 1: Denying the Problem

When a hospital is in denial, its management and board have difficulty recognizing that they are responsible for the hospital's problems. They cite external reasons why things are not going well and why the hospital continues to lose money. (Someone or something beyond executive control is always to blame.) Typical excuses offered to explain productivity and cost-control shortfalls in hospitals include the following:

- "My patients are sicker."
- "Medicare isn't fair."
- "The other departments aren't doing their jobs."
- "The doctors won't cooperate."
- "It's not my job."

Not accepting the responsibility for problems creates a self-fulfilling prophecy: disaster is on the horizon and nothing can be done about it. During the denial phase, management typically only makes changes that are forced on them by external organizations (for example, the Health Care Financing Administration or the Joint Commission on Accreditation of Healthcare Organizations). Unsolved issues cause more problems, and the absence of an organizationwide problem-solving process creates even more problems.

The chart shown in figure 2-1 illustrates the differences in mind-set between a successful hospital and a failing hospital. The unsuccessful hospital is a reactive organization. With its external view of problems, the hospital makes few changes until an individual or an organization with greater authority, control, or power dictates that they must. Then, with great exasperation, management shifts its attention to solving its problems.

The shortcomings of this organizational behavior are obvious. The hospital often focuses on alleviating symptoms instead of remedying underlying problems. As a result, another set of symptoms eventually surfaces, either immediately or in the very near future, and because management has diverted the majority of its attention to this one crisis, other problems arise, are ignored, and then grow into problems of comparable proportions. Soon, one of these other problems will become a crisis, not because the problem has gotten worse, but because an outside authority has brought the problem to the hospital's attention. The hospital that continues to take this reactive posture is in danger of financial failure and eventual closure.

During the denial phase, proactive improvement is seldom considered, although *proactive* may be used as a buzzword among managers of an unsuccessful hospital. Everyone rushes to react to "supplies costing too much" or "payroll being too high." As the problems mount, the areas that are running relatively smoothly do not get the management attention they need and deserve. Soon, morale declines and performance deteriorates. And, as management attacks morale and performance problems, other problems arise as a result of management's solutions. Management only notices the new problems when the problems reach proportions large enough to qualify as the new crisis of the day.

Figure 2-1. Perspectives on Change

	Successful Hospital	Unsuccessful Hospital
Perspective	Internal	External
Most common pronoun(s)	"We"	"They," "me"
Change posture	Proactive	Reactive

Personalities become a key issue as management takes an emotional approach to problems during the denial phase. Management tries to find who, rather than what, is responsible for the problem. Sometimes, the result is firings that do not make a lot of sense. Other workers, often the more skillful workers, might become disillusioned and quit. When individuals within an organization are singled out, general problems are not solved, and real improvement does not take place.

When looking for who has caused a problem, the unsuccessful hospital uses pronouns differently from a successful hospital. As a problem arises, it is easy to find the cause. *They* did it. Terms are used constantly such as *my people* and "if you could only get *them* to do *their* job, then *you* wouldn't be coming to *me* about this." More progressive hospitals generally use a different pronoun—**we.** Looking at problems in terms of how *we* can do better will generally lead to more effective solutions (even when *we* had nothing to do with creating the problem). It is surprising the difference a pronoun makes in attitudes.

Hospitals that use "we" tend to look at problems internally. If "we" have a problem, then everyone has a part in solving it. Employees worry less about presenting a problem when they know their colleagues will not be singled out for blame. Using this internal perspective helps a hospital identify and solve a problem before it reaches the crisis level. To the hospital in denial, this concept "sounds good on paper, but just can't work in the real world."

Probably most puzzling during the denial phase is that everyone is working hard. Work is simply not getting done in a manner that meets departmental or institutional requirements. Unfortunately, management does not know or believe that many of the problems exist. Hospital managers should ask themselves questions like these: Is the hospital in the denial phase? What pronouns are being used? Are board members suffering from denial as well?

Hospital operations may have to "bottom out," or some trauma may have to occur before management realizes its behavior must change. Malpractice suits may increase. Physicians might start to leave the hospital in record numbers. The hospital's community image may begin to deteriorate. Once warning signs appear, management begins "sobering up," the next phase.

Phase 2: Sobering Up

When the sobering-up phase begins, the hospital starts to realize that some costs can be reduced and that productivity can be improved. Typically, areas in which costs appear to be high are listed, and teams are formed to find methods to reduce costs. Department contests designed to spark employee enthusiasm are created, and budgetary charts begin to show improvement. The investigation results, however, usually only lead to short-term remedies. Nearsighted managers reason, "We don't have time to go into long-term solutions. We've got patients to see, medical records to complete, claims to file, accounts to collect, and trouble just trying to stay alive as a hospital."

Although problems are being recognized, management often underestimates the nature and extent of the problems. Often while the management is sobering up, there is a tendency to think, after problem-solving energy has been expended, that problems are getting worse instead of better. In fact, the hospital is starting to uncover problems that have always existed, but were never noticed before. Additionally, some problems that had been "fixed" during this phase begin to surface again because of the short-term approach to the remedy.

As the hospital seems to regress, management may want to rethink its approach to problem solving. However, the increased surfacing of problems must be recognized as part of the improvement process. Management needs to realize that while attacking problems, the process for creating long-term solutions must improve, without losing sight of the hospital's objectives.

Rethinking the approach to problem solving is a critical point in the hospital's progress in developing cost-reduction strategies. It is easy, in this time of reevaluation, for the administration and the board to become discouraged. A change in management may occur, or cost-containment initiatives may be labeled "ineffective." If either of these situations occurs, the hospital will quickly slip back into the denial stage.

Which direction the hospital takes at this point may well depend on the hospital's informal leaders, as well as the rest of the workers. Employees below the management level can offer much to the entire cost-containment process. Due to their daily "hands-on" work, these front-line employees know more about every aspect of the hospital's operation than do managers. These employees recognize that without improved performance, the hospital cannot continue to exist. If managers can effectively communicate to workers that greater efficiency is necessary to improve the quality of care being delivered, the hospital can move forward in the process. Achieving full staff participation in the problem-solving process is the critical step in becoming a "born-again" cost-controlling hospital.

Phase 3: Being Born Again

A thoughtful and farsighted approach to problem resolution is the telltale sign of a born-again hospital. Problems are identified and discussed openly, focusing on processes instead of blaming individuals. Problems are elaborated with facts, not opinions. Investigators analyze causes and effects, and several solutions are generated before deciding which one to implement. The first solution to be implemented should be selected with care. The hospital's first improvement project must be one that has a high probability of success, with easily tracked results.

During this first improvement project, workers become excited as they participate in the process. It is important that this excitement be maintained beyond involvement in this initial project. Management must continuously reassure employees that every future problem can be solved by using this method. To keep employees interested and motivated the following strategies should be considered:

- Handpicking employees who have good attitudes and the ability to successfully complete the tasks at hand
- Choosing an initial problem, something that most likely can be solved in a short period of time
- Conveying the fact that every project takes time in planning, execution, and improvement and may even exhaust its usefulness at some point
- Giving the project team time to fully understand the objectives and components of each task to be performed
- Having a measurable and attainable goal for the team

There will still be problems during this born-again phase, but workers will start to identify cost control areas, work patterns, and opportunities for greater efficiency. Most important, improvement will occur, and employees will generally feel that things are changing for the better.

Phase 4: Feeling Wiser but Cautious

Although the born-again phase may inspire confidence and pride, the hospital must next focus on maintaining cost containment. This phase is the time to develop new goals for the hospital, ways to do things better. The following attitudes are displayed frequently:

- Any problems that appear can be quickly and easily solved.
- The hospital can accomplish any task, no matter how difficult.
- Employees and medical staff feel they are working well together and can do little wrong.
- The hospital runs like a well-oiled machine.

The worst thing managers and administrators can do at this point is to take their employees, or the seemingly untroubled state of the hospital, for granted. They may be tempted to delegate problem solving to support staff, allowing managers and administrators to concentrate on new programs and services. Confident managers and administrators may feel little need to ponder staffing, budget, and physician profile variances. But if they relax their problem-solving efforts, they can fall right back into denial. To avoid repeating old patterns, a no-nonsense approach to *variances* must become a daily practice and corporate culture.

Phase 5: Becoming a Serious Cost Container

Very few hospitals ever reach this final phase, although because of its size, a smaller hospital has the best chance. When a hospital becomes a serious cost container, it boasts realistic operational outcomes and rarely incurs significant cost problems. The basic mind-set is that waste should not occur. Even in this phase, however, basic trends must be continuously monitored. A "we're on top of the world, now let's stay there!" organizational attitude needs to be adopted. With daily operations running well and variances rarely occurring, the hospital's challenge shifts to adjusting and responding to the continuously changing regulatory environment. With some irony, hospital managers may note that their confidence level in this final phase of cost control is as high as it had been in the denial phase. These five phases of cost containment show that ignorance is not bliss.

The Creativity Cycle for Positioning the Hospital for Change

As the saying goes, "If you've seen one hospital, you've seen one hospital." It is difficult to determine the specific needs of a particular hospital. Hospitals with fewer than 100 beds, however, typically do not need highly sophisticated cost-management systems. Smaller hospitals need a good budgeting process (discussed in chapter 3) and an environment that allows creative development of appropriate and efficient methods of delivering health care services. Reducing costs requires change, and that change must be conceived, accepted, and executed by the people who work in and with the hospital.

It is a fact of life that organizations are resistant to change. "If it ain't broke, don't fix it," staff will complain, "We've never done it this way before." The protests against change seem endless, but people are not resisting the innovation itself as much as having to personally change. Much of this resistance can be avoided by:

- Involving employees in designing the change
- Explaining changes to employees early and thoroughly
- Demonstrating the benefit of the change

• Not criticizing the previous method (allowing the employees to critically evaluate past outcomes)

Successful management does not depend on finding the final solution for every problem; if it did, managers would not be necessary. Despite employee creativity and operational efficiency, problems will continue to arise. Success depends on effective and continuous improvement. A tool called the creativity cycle can be used to resolve problems, budget variances, and other deviations from standard operations. With the tool, performance and productivity are likely to improve continuously.

There are seven steps to the creativity cycle:

1. Identify the problem (or opportunity to improve).
2. Gather the facts.
3. Analyze the facts.
4. Identify possible solutions.
5. Select the preferred solution.
6. Implement the preferred solution.
7. Monitor the improved performance.

Creativity should be examined one step at a time.

Step 1: Identify the Problem

Bob and Jim went fishing together one Saturday. Unfortunately, the fish were not biting. Each saw this as a problem. Bob wondered, "How do we get the fish to start biting?" Jim worried, "How do I convince my family I actually went fishing?" The same circumstances can often lead individuals to view a problem in different ways. Every person views a problem as a conclusion, based on how they frame the situation. Perceptions are often colored by past experiences. If people are to solve a problem, they must see it the same way.

If a staffing report lists nursing as performing with only 75 percent productivity, the problem may be interpreted differently by administrators than by nurse managers. Administration may judge the problem to be too many nurses on staff. Nursing might view the problem as additional tasks being performed by nurses that are not considered to be standard nursing care. The solution may be recognition that both parties are correct, and if lower-paid, easier-to-recruit personnel are used to perform the additional tasks, nurse staffing needs will be reduced. Long-term improvements in productivity can only be made when people interpret problems the same way. To help staff view a problem similarly and define a problem accurately, stating the objectives and explaining the problem are helpful.

Stating the Objectives

The number of existing problems to solve is sometimes overwhelming. By looking at problems in terms of stated organizational objectives, one can select which problems to solve first, and in what priority. Problems and opportunities for improvement must be considered in terms of hospital and departmental objectives. Often a great deal of time is spent solving problems that do not help achieve organizational objectives. If time is being wasted on problems that do not help achieve objectives, reevaluation is needed for either the types of problems being attacked or the stated objectives.

Efforts should be concentrated in a direction that allows one to take advantage of the current hospital environment. The very circumstances that at first appear to be obstacles to success can very often be instrumental to success.

It is important to establish the nature of the problem, where it exists, who is involved, when it occurs, and how it occurs. Memory or personal opinion is not reliable when examining a problem. The whole problem must be seen as it happens, not as framed by another individual. If the problem is difficult to observe, accounts of the problem from workers with firsthand experience should be gathered.

Explaining the Problem

Basically, there are two types of problems: those identified by someone else and those that are self-identified. As discussed in the phases of cost containment, there can be significant differences in the way problems are identified. In the denial phase, hospital management rarely identifies its own problems; for serious cost containers, cost problems rarely surface outside the department in which they occur. Cost problems are contained because, as the hospital passes through the phases of cost containment, it becomes more skillful at monitoring its performance and using the creativity cycle to correct variances, develop new ideas, and advance performance standards. Returning to the above example of underutilization in the nursing department, a way of stating the problem might be, "The hospital's contractual adjustments are 25 percent higher than budget."

Step 2: Get the Facts

The first step in the fact-finding process is to review or develop departmental or hospital objectives. Often "great" solutions are discovered that do not actually solve the problem at hand. If a solution does not support the realization of objectives, then the wrong problem has been solved. If departmental or hospital objectives are unclear or unknown, then that is a more pressing problem. In gathering facts about targeted problems, one must remain open-minded about change, make sure the facts are being dealt with, see the problem firsthand, and perform a work distribution study.

Remaining Open-Minded about Change

More than likely, "the way we have always done it" in the hospital, from replacing hips to changing bed sheets, can probably be done more efficiently or effectively. Managers within the hospital must sincerely feel that they have a continuous responsibility to make improvements. If an area has not been improved over the past 12 months, an opportunity is probably being missed.

Making Sure that Facts Are Being Discussed

When an employee presents an issue as a fact, the sources of their information and how they arrived at their calculations should be questioned (inquisitively, not accusingly). Hearsay and opinion should not be stated as fact. A co-worker could possibly act on a dubious "fact" and choose an unwise course of action.

Witnessing the Problem Firsthand

It is important that a problem be witnessed firsthand and an analysis made in a similar manner. Employees affected by the problem should be interviewed. As has been noted, people see the same problem differently based on their own past experiences.

It is helpful to use charts and graphs in gathering and displaying facts about a problem. Besides their analytic value, charts and graphs allow the presentation of facts in a clear and concise manner. Charts and graphs also help investigators studying the problem to see things the same way. Finally, when a solution has been developed, charts and graphs can be used for training personnel in the new method.

Performing a Work Distribution Study

A great number of facts are needed in order to improve productivity. One method to gather the facts is to use a work distribution study. A work distribution study should answer questions such as: What work is being done? Who is doing it? How long should it take? By answering such questions, management can show whether, and to what extent, work is being evenly distributed. The activities that consume the most time can be identified. The study can determine how often clinical employees are being used to perform clinical work and how much time they spend completing clerical work. The study can determine whether the performance standards include how much time is being spent on each activity. A work distribution study can also determine which job responsibilities are not being completed or are being completed by expensive, temporary agency help.

A work distribution study can be conducted not only by managers, but by any employee. A daily record is kept by each employee showing how much time is being spent on each task being performed. At the end of a selected period of time, the employees can determine the average amount of time it takes to perform each task and summarize their findings. The supervisor can then list the time it takes to perform each departmental task and the tasks' relationships to each other. If managers take the time to explain the work distribution study process, the study's importance, and the fact that it is the *work* that is being studied, not the *workers*, a high level of cooperation and reporting accuracy over the course of the study is likely.

Important to consider, however, when planning a work distribution study is the substantial amount of time involved. In administering a study, managers and administrators must be prepared for the probability that the information will not be complete or accurate because it is being done by employees who are overburdened by their routine work responsibilities. It should not be surprising if department heads request additional staffing just so the study can be completed. Work distribution studies are not always the best way to obtain reasonably accurate data.

The facts related to a stated problem are certain to reveal information toward the development of possible solutions. Facts associated with the problem identified at the end of step 1 may include some similar to the following examples:

- The hospital's Medicare denial rate has increased by 15 percent over the past year.
- The hospital's only precertification review for Medicare and Medicaid cases is done by the admissions clerk.
- The organisms responsible in 9 out of 10 pneumonia cases reviewed are not being specified.
- The length of stay has increased 15 percent overall and 25 percent for pneumonia cases.
- All utilization review is being performed retrospectively by the medical record director.
- Discharge planning does not begin at the time of admission.

Step 3: Analyze the Facts

Once the facts have been gathered and listed, the facts should be subjected to a logical sequence of questions that will lead to more efficient solutions. This sequence consists of questions about the what, why, where, when, who, and how, followed by the analysis of trends and the creation of a fact analysis.

Asking What, Why, Where, When, Who, and How

Analyzing what is being done, why it is being done, and what else could be done in addition will help eliminate unnecessary parts of a job. By examining a job's location (where each task is being done, why it is being done there, and identifying if it could be done anywhere else), its sequence (when each task is done, why it is done at that time, must it be done at that time, and when else might it be done), and the person associated with the job (who is doing it, why that person does the job, who might be able to complete the job faster, better, cheaper), solutions may become obvious that result in the combining of two or more tasks, a more cost-effective assignment of duties, and a better flow of the process for completing the task. Finally, analyzing how the task is performed and why it is performed in that way may lead to improved or simplified execution of the tasks' components.

Analyzing Trends

A key component to identifying work problems and separating facts from opinions is trend analysis. A trend is a general pattern or direction of activity that can be determined through comparing information over a period of time. An example of a trend analysis would be a comparison of supply costs per procedure that indicates supply costs are rising by 2 percent per month.

Department managers can identify trends by plotting monthly financial and operational results over a period of time. Budget variances (explained in chapter 3) can be plotted each month to provide a graphic representation of budget trends during a specific period of time. Table 2-1 illustrates how trends indicate a pattern of direct expense variances for a radiology department. In this example, the expense variance increases as utilization decreases. These historical trends not only help identify potential opportunities for immediate improvement, but they also help predict the future. Continued monitoring of test volumes, for instance, can be used to predict the volume of next year's tests.

Table 2-1. Sample Trend Analysis: XYZ Hospital Radiology Department

		Months			
	1	2	3	4	5
Tests	2150	1895	2351	2126	1995
Revenue	$86,000	$75,000	$91,000	$85,000	$79,000
Direct expense[a]	$1,200	$2,200	$0	$1,500	$1,900

[a]Figures represent variances beyond tolerance levels.

For trend analysis to be useful, it is important to identify a trend's cause. The trend itself is usually only a symptom. In table 2-1, the variance may indicate that the hospital is not adjusting staffing based on changes in volumes. Or the variance may imply that physicians are ordering more costly tests than what are being reported in common procedural terminology (CPT) codes for payment. Or the variance might indicate that the hospital is not capturing all the charges when certain tests are performed. Problem solving helps correct variances by attacking the problem's cause. Predictions will become important when it is understood whether the cause of the pattern will be a factor in the future.

Trends are most valuable when plotted on monthly and year-to-date intervals. Monthly and year-to-year performance can then be easily compared. Decisions based on these plotted trends must take into account both improving and deteriorating trends in utilization, operational statistics, costs, revenues, operating profits, and departmental contribution.

In analyzing trends and prioritizing improvement opportunities, management should identify to what extent reported performance will be allowed to vary from the targeted amount (either over or under the targeted amount) before recommending extensive study for improvement. This variance is called a tolerance level and is usually expressed as a percentage of a budgeted amount or developed standard. Table 2-1 illustrates that only months 1, 2, 4, and 5 experienced variances in excess of tolerance levels.

Creating a Fact Analysis

Careful trend analysis should reveal several facts about a problem. These facts in turn reveal the causes of particular variances and lead to corrective measures. Analyzing the facts listed at the end of step 2 leads to the emergence of several ideas.

Medicare denial rate has increased with precertification review for Medicare and Medicaid cases performed by the admissions clerk alone. The denial rate can be explained by several facts associated with the hospital's pre-certification procedures. If an admissions clerk performs the precertification screening, the hospital may miss the chance for additional nurse or physician case review, helpful to ensure that clinical criteria are met. Often, through consultation with a physician's office, the patient might be redirected to an outpatient setting and avoid Medicare denial. In other cases, a physician's office can prompt for more appropriate documentation, resulting in a diagnosis that qualifies a patient for admission. The end result would be identification of a more cost-effective treatment path, as well as a reduction of charges during the patient's length of stay.

Organisms are not specified on 9 out of 10 pneumonia cases reviewed, and length of stay has increased 15 percent overall and 25 percent for pneumonia cases. Usually, a specific organism (*Klebsiella, Streptococcus, Staphylococcus,* and so forth) can be identified in over 10 percent of pneumonia cases. Identification of an organism may enable an attending physician to prescribe a specific antibiotic to treat the organism. A specified antibiotic is often less costly and more effective than a global antibiotic and leads to lower drug costs and shorter lengths of inpatient stay. Specifying an organism also qualifies the hospital for a higher-paying diagnostic-related group (DRG).

All utilization review is performed retrospectively by the medical record director. A patient can be managed much more effectively if the case is reviewed during the length of stay (concurrently). If a patient has been admitted without meeting the payer's criteria for admission, utilization review can correct this problem early in the stay. Identification of specific entries into a patient's record (such as the specified organism) can be brought to the attention of the physician immediately, allowing correction of inappropriate case treatment plans.

Discharge planning does not begin at the time of admission. Starting discharge planning at admission can reduce a patient's length of stay. Postponing discharge planning until the end of a patient's stay often unnecessarily prolongs the discharge process. Concurrent discharge planning is especially important for patients who will probably need to be discharged to a nursing home. Nursing home beds in close proximity to the hospital are often not available, and alternative sites must be considered. Knowing a hospital's policies and attitude toward issuing "termination of benefits" notification to guarantors also plays an important role in timely discharge planning.

Step 4: Identify Possible Solutions

Completing step 4 requires creativity. Once problems have been clearly identified, and supporting facts have been studied, it is time to shift attention back to hospital and departmental objectives. Many managers fail during this phase because they try to find excuses instead of solutions to their problems. Other managers do not allow departments to reach their potential because problem solving is the goal, rather than the meeting of objectives. Staff creativity will substantially improve once the focus returns to objectives.

It may be tempting to obsessively struggle against inflexible conditions, such as those imposed by health care regulations. Creative management requires innovative thought in the face of challenges. Instead of worrying about the consequences of seemingly unsolvable problems ("I'll lose my job," "the physicians will stop admitting patients," and so forth), the creative manager analyzes how a difficult situation can help the hospital reach its objectives.

At this point, another account of how creativity leads to cost-effective improvements may be helpful. For example, a hospital experienced higher costs because of the extensive use of contract nursing. Initially, the management team framed the problem as a nursing shortage problem. The team spent enormous amounts of money on advertisements in the local newspaper to attract new nurses, with little success. Management stated the problem as "what am I going to do about our nursing shortage?" They did not arrive at any reasonable solutions until they began to decide "how are we going to live with the nursing shortage?" This rephrased question inspired the following ideas:

- Cross-train all nurses to at least one other hospital department.
- Rotate existing nurses to other shifts to redistribute the work load.
- Develop an internal nursing pool by recruiting nurses from the city and pay a per-diem rate higher than the hourly rate, but lower than agency rates.
- Persuade other small hospitals in the area to join in the development of the nursing pool.
- Reassign rudimentary nursing duties, freeing nurses to perform skilled-level tasks and hiring ward clerks and orderlies to perform clerical tasks and patient transportation.

Because management rephrased the nursing shortage question, innovative solutions appeared. Management used perceived obstacles to the hospital's advantage. A nursing shortage became a nursing pool.

Step 5: Select the Preferred Solution

After listing all possible solutions, an evaluation process should be used to select the preferred solution. Sometimes managers will doubt that they have chosen the preferred solution. In this case, managers should not be afraid to retrace steps in the problem-solving cycle. More data may have to be gathered. It may be determined that the problem has not been fully described. A few short experiments may be necessary to better evaluate each of the solutions (usually more solutions can be added to the list as the result of these experiments). Once the preferred solution is determined, the solution should be displayed in the form of a chart so that everyone can visualize the solution in the same way.

Step 6: Implement the Preferred Solution

Common sense dictates that in order to improve things, one must implement the preferred solution. Yet poor execution of a solution is the second-biggest area of failure in the creativity cycle (after identifying the problem). Implementing a solution starts with proper planning. Component tasks must be clearly defined, responsibility for their execution should be assigned to specific individuals, and a timetable with completion dates must be established. Each task should be clearly associated with the solution's objectives. Both the solution's objectives and the component tasks must be fully discussed with everyone involved in implementing the improvements.

Step 7: Monitor Improvements

To fully determine whether a problem has been solved, results of the improvement efforts must be monitored. A method of recording results should be developed. A review of results helps identify whether the problem was completely solved, whether the right problem was solved, and whether other problems have appeared during the problem-solving process. While efforts to resolve one problem are under way, other problems may arise. Identifying and solving problems will be a never-ending task for the hospital that wants to improve continuously.

The Budget as a Management Tool

A good understanding of the problem-solving process is essential to positioning a hospital for change. This understanding also sets the stage for using the hospital's financial budget as a very powerful tool. The hospital's budget utilizes trends and reports variances from expected standards. In so doing, the budget helps the hospital identify problems and monitor the effect of improvement efforts. The budget process, and how this process can be used as a management tool, are discussed in the next chapter.

Reference

1. Crosby, P. *Quality Is Free: The Art of Making Quality Certain.* New York
   City: New American Library, 1979.

Chapter 3

Making the Budget Work

A budget is simply a plan, and it should not be burdened with negative connotations. It is a strategy expressed in dollars and cents.
Adjusting hospital services to realistically meet community health care
needs while lowering the costs of providing those services are the most
significant challenges facing a small hospital. The exemplary manager
should use his or her budget as a mandate for meeting these challenges.

A well-designed budget is an expression of the hospital's goals, a
method of performance evaluation, and a tool for communication and
coordination. Most important, a well-designed budget forces managers
to plan for the future. For smaller hospitals, the budget is the hospital's
cost-accounting system. Smaller hospitals have a relatively simple
management structure and a large portion of fixed costs due to low
patient volumes. Such hospitals often fail to recognize these important
qualities, and as a result budgets take more time to develop, do not
realistically reflect planned operations, and almost instantly become
obsolete—a waste of time, energy, money, and opportunity.

Hospital budgets are usually prepared on an annual basis and should
be analyzed monthly for variances and adjustments. Budgets should be
adjusted on a monthly basis to reflect internal and external changes outside the manager's control. However, when changes and variances occur
within a manager's sphere of influence, performance should be adjusted
immediately.

151,909

Budgets and Budgeting

Budgeting differs from actual budgets because budgeting includes controlling mechanisms as well as planning mechanisms. The budgeting
process is a useful tool in helping a hospital achieve budgetary goals
through frequent comparisons of actual and budgeted amounts. Monitoring discrepancies between budgeted and actual amounts is the most

important step in containing costs in a smaller hospital. Investigations of variances and corrective actions help keep a hospital on track toward meeting its goals.

Budgeting comparisons are usually made on a monthly basis. Monthly comparisons help a hospital to "flex" its budget, addressing costs more appropriately as utilization varies from forecasted levels. Hospital management is then able to analyze costs relative to actual volumes of service.

Goals and Objectives

Goals and objectives are extremely important in creating the budget. Goals are set during the planning stages, along with strategies to accomplish those goals. The planning process should include a forecast of service units, revenues, and costs for the next fiscal year. These forecasts are the hospital's goals. Control of budget variances requires measurement of how well the hospital is performing in light of its goals, and then taking corrective actions when significant variances are discovered.

Because goals and objectives are important to the planning process, they require concrete definitions. A *goal* is a general statement of intent that reflects the direction and priorities of the hospital. An *objective* is a specific statement that clearly describes what, when, and how something is going to be accomplished. An objective also provides standards for measuring performance. In the planning process, objectives must be realistic and challenging. To meet control requirements, objectives must also be measurable.

Action Plans

An action plan should be developed by each department director, including stated goals and objectives, as well as the specific tasks to be completed. The planned tasks should include target completion dates. With each task, a responsible agent should be assigned to ensure that the task is completed. The checklist in figure 3-1 was designed to help the manager make sure the action plan is complete.

Figure 3-1.   Action Plan Checklist

_____ Have objectives been developed to support an overall goal?
_____ Does the plan relate to the accomplishment of a stated objective?
_____ Is the plan realistic for the department?
_____ Is there a method to measure the result?
_____ Has a completion date been assigned to each task?
_____ Is there a responsible agent assigned for each task?

Once an action plan has been implemented, it must be continuously updated. The plan should highlight tasks that are completed and any adjustments that need to be made. The budget itself, through reporting of variance in actual performance, will provide the most critical monitoring information of the plan. The budget indicates to the manager whether objectives are being met and should direct the manager to potential problem areas in each department. Any resultant budget or objective adjustments should then be reflected in the action plan.

Quantifying Goals and Objectives

Quantifying goals and objectives usually are the result of problem solving. Once the solution to a problem is identified, a manager should be ready to estimate the solution's effect in terms of statistics or dollars. These statistics and dollars are not arbitrary; they are based on collected data and become the meterstick for determining whether objectives have been met. The more specific an objective, the easier it is to quantify.

Figure 3-2 is an example of a developed goal, with corresponding objectives and associated tasks. The second and third objectives in figure 3-2 can be used as staff exercises to develop sample tasks. In the space provided, staff should add the quantification components of statistics and dollar amounts as shown in objective 1. These examples should be a springboard to develop future departmental goals and objectives.

Cost Management and the Budget

The budget is a smaller hospital's most effective cost management system. Because smaller hospitals are primarily focused on maintaining utilization and controlling costs on a broad basis, a cost management system must provide information to help a hospital manage its resources appropriately. An effective cost management system should help a smaller hospital:

- Improve profits (reserves) and cash flow
- Improve departmental performance
- Analyze departmental work flows
- Develop bidding strategies for managed care

Historically, controlling costs has been a strategic issue more troubling to smaller hospitals than to larger hospitals. Smaller hospitals have a larger portion of fixed costs because they must provide services with lower volumes and limited access to skilled labor. Thus, the amount of time it takes to provide a chest X ray, compared to a foot X ray, is of

Figure 3-2. Sample Goal, Objectives, and Tasks

Goal: To reduce operating expenses in patient care areas by 6 percent

Objective 1: Develop cross-sharing system of nurses between med/surg, emergency, ICU, surgery, and recovery, reducing 4 FTEs and $96,000 in salaries and $45,000 in temporary nursing service expenses.

Tasks	Agent(s)	Due Date
Review credentials and experience levels of each nursing staff member	Director of nursing	June 21
Identify task force	Director of nursing	June 28
Convene task force	Director of nursing	July 1
Develop cross-sharing matrix	Task force	Aug. 31
Train nurses on process	Task force	Sept. 15
Train nurses in expanded functions	Supervisors	Sept. 16–15
Initiate system	Director of nursing	Jan. 2

Objective 2: Reduce non–patient-related tasks being performed by nursing personnel.

Tasks	Agent(s)	Due Date

Objective 3: Develop treatment protocols for the hospital's top 10 DRGs in gross revenue.

Tasks	Agent(s)	Due Date

little consequence in a smaller hospital. The important issues are how to use staff time efficiently when radiography personnel are not performing any tasks; how to streamline work flow, distribute scarce labor skills, retain and recruit qualified staff, and effectively cross-train personnel; and how to maintain utilization volumes and appropriately use available facilities. An effective budget and budgeting process helps a hospital do these things.

Forecasting for Units of Service

Forecasting the level of utilization at a hospital is an important part of the planning process. Budgeted revenues, staffing costs, and variable costs are driven by forecasts. A budget can only be valid if the hospital selects units of service that appropriately relate to its outputs (department production), resources (direct costs), and applicable revenues.

As hospital caseloads continue to experience significant shifts to the outpatient setting, forecasts will present an increasing challenge. This transition is occurring at different rates for different hospitals. Some smaller hospitals report that 20 percent of their revenue comes from outpatient services, but this figure is as high as 70 percent in others. With the continued growth in managed care initiatives, more stringent Medicare admitting criteria, and continued advances in medical technology, the challenge will be to forecast how fast this transformation will take place in each service area. It will be extremely important for managers to closely monitor these trends and to adjust their budgets accordingly.

In addition, it will be important that communication channels within the hospital remain open. A budget should reflect any service additions or deletions at the hospital. The budget should also consider the effect of physicians joining or leaving the medical staff. For example, if additional physicians in certain specialties are being recruited and are anticipated to arrive in the community within the budget year, departmental inpatient and outpatient forecasts could be significantly affected.

To develop a budget, utilization must be estimated for each department. This is done by forecasting units of service such as adjusted patient days, laboratory tests (or relative value units), emergency or clinic visits, radiology tests, meals served, surgery minutes, and so forth. Patient days are usually forecast first, which then allows other departments whose activities are driven by census to forecast their revenues.

Most hospitals, especially smaller hospitals, calculate patient days factoring outpatient utilization through a unit of service called adjusted average daily census. Adjusted average daily census is calculated by multiplying a hospital's average daily census for a certain period by an adjustment factor, which is the ratio of gross patient revenue to gross inpatient revenue. Figure 3-3 demonstrates one such calculation.

Figure 3-3. Sample Calculation for Adjusted Average Daily Census

Given:

Hospital gross revenue   = $12,000,000

Hospital inpatient revenue   = $8,000,000

Hospital annual patient days =   3,650

(1) Compute average daily census

     3,650 ÷ 365 = 10 patients

(2) Compute adjusted average daily census

     10 × ($12,000,000 ÷ $8,000,000) = 15 patients

New standards are being developed that reflect case management–oriented care. A case weight-adjusted stay, recognizing a unit of service, will most likely replace average daily census as the common relative value unit. This value will consider inpatient standards based on the time a patient is in the hospital and the severity of illness associated with the stay. This standard will more closely reflect a payment system based on diagnosis-related groups (DRGs).

In budget forecasting, utilization levels are predicted in terms of departmental units of service for the next fiscal year. The following terms are examples of departmental units of service:

Department	Units of Service
Medical/surgical nursing	Medical/surgical adjusted patient days
Operating room	Surgery minutes
Central supply	Total adjusted patient days
Radiology	Radiology tests
Emergency	Emergency department visits

Once those predictions are made, revenues and costs can be forecast. Ideally, it should be possible to acquire valuable information to generate forecasts from the hospital's strategic plan. Unfortunately, many hospitals still do not have a strategic plan, and others do not update their plan annually. (Readers may wish to refer to two 1989 publications from the American Hospital Association: *Strategic Planning Workbook* and *A Prelude to Strategic Planning: Making Your Organization and Community Fit for Success.*)

When predicting units of service, the following points must be considered:

- *Historical trends:* It is important to examine downward and upward shifts in inpatient and outpatient service. Management should try to predict future activity by identifying the causes of change. What has been the effect of the regulatory environment? What has been the effect of changing physician patterns?

- *Anticipated physician utilization:* Predicting utilization requires communication with the medical staff throughout the year. Management must know which practices are expanding, which are winding down, and which specialists are receiving referrals from primary care physicians. How will these trends change in the future?

- *New or expanded service impact:* The budget should accommodate increases in utilization from planned, new, or recently expanded programs. Forecasts should also reflect any potential utilization trade-offs from new services that will cause reduced levels of utilization elsewhere. Will new procedures replace the need for other procedures? Will the opening of a new clinic reduce the volume of patients in the emergency department?

- *Other internal and external utilization factors:* Various factors such as recent and anticipated changes in facility operations, physician behavior and recruitment, and regulatory changes should be reviewed. For example, how will outpatient and inpatient activity change when a physical therapist resigns? When is a physical therapy replacement expected?

Patient days are usually the first unit of measure to be addressed in the forecast of service utilization. Patient days are initially considered because most other units are gauged from inpatient activity. Even though outpatient activity continues to increase, many hospitals continue to track activity levels based on inpatient activity. Nevertheless, hospitals need to begin shifting their mode of tracking to more appropriately reflect actual departmental activity. If a hospital has enough volume in certain departments to support utilization derived primarily from inpatient volumes (for example, the intensive care unit, obstetrics and gynecology services), then forecasts based on predictions of the number of patient days will continue to be appropriate for those departments. Overall, department-specific units of service is the key to forecasting revenues, staffing requirements, and other variable and semivariable costs.

The Department-Level Budget

Using the budget as a management tool is a matter of responsibility and accountability. It is the CEO's responsibility to ensure hospitalwide cost containment, including the development and maintenance of the hospital's budget. An accurately planned, properly coordinated, and closely controlled budget is the most important financial management tool available to the smaller hospital. The actual development and execution of the budget is accomplished by each department manager, who, after attending physicians, have the most control over reducing hospital costs. Although a CEO can never delegate his or her responsibilities, it is critical to make each department accountable for meeting standards stated in the budget.

Cost-control concepts will change significantly during the current era of health care reform. Hospitals have traditionally looked at reducing costs in light of the units of service delivered. At the same time, the hospital's marketing objectives have been to increase units of service. Health care reform initiatives will create incentives designed to alter providers' objectives, so that access to health care services is expanded but the actual units of service decline. The end result should be an alignment of the providers' cost-control objectives with the cost-control objectives of those who pay for the care. (This reform strategy is discussed further in chapter 7.)

Much of a hospital's success in controlling costs will come from changing physician utilization behavior through collaboration between hospital management and medical staff. By exploring new outpatient and home health treatment options, which focus on early detection and management of chronic illness, the overall cost of providing health care should be reduced. Once the strategic direction of physician utilization is set and patient treatment adheres to specific protocols, the department manager has the most control over costs in the hospital. In smaller hospitals, the best tool available to the department manager for planning, monitoring, and controlling costs is the department-level budget.

The Differences between Costs and Expenses

To develop a department-level budget, a few terms must be defined. The terms *cost* and *expense* are often used interchangeably; however, each term has a distinct meaning. *Cost* can be defined as what was paid for some good, service, or other benefit. Accountants describe the cost of an item as what is paid to acquire it. *Expense* is how the cost is reported on income statements and budgets. Expense refers to the costs matched to the revenues that the costs generate.

An item is a cost before it becomes an expense. If a case of surgical gowns is purchased, one can refer to the cost of the gowns. If the gowns have not yet been used on patients, an accountant could not consider this cost to be an expense. Additionally, a cost can only be an expense in the period in which the revenues associated with that cost are recorded. Until a cost becomes an expense, it is generally treated as an asset (such as inventory).

Types of Costs and Expenses

Different types of costs and expenses behave differently in the budget process. For managers to budget effectively, they must know the difference between fixed, variable, and semivariable costs and expenses. It is also necessary to discriminate among the various types of expenses.

Fixed Costs and Expenses

Fixed costs and expenses remain the same, regardless of any changes in hospital activity. Fixed rentals, administrative and marketing services, and educational programs are examples of fixed costs. On a per-unit basis, fixed costs and expenses fluctuate as volumes change. This quality is important in analyzing smaller hospital performance. The relatively high fixed cost of staffing in smaller hospitals can dramatically skew accepted operational ratios such as full-time equivalents (FTEs) per occupied bed. Fixed costs are also called periodic costs because they are associated with periods of time, not with the rendering of services.

Variable Costs and Expenses

Variable costs and expenses change with fluctuations of activity levels. Medical fees and supplies commonly represent variable costs and expenses. Any increase in volume affects variable costs and expenses. However, on a per-unit basis, variable costs and expenses remain static as volumes change. The following is an example of how variable costs are calculated: If radiology film costs $6,708 for one month and total radiology tests for the same month number 2,080, then the variable expense for that month is $6,708 divided by 2,080 tests, or $3.23 per test.

Semivariable Costs and Expenses

Semivariable costs and expenses vary, but not proportionately with volumes. Often, a portion of semivariable costs, such as salaries, can be treated as fixed costs, while the remaining costs for that area are variable. More specifically, some salary costs and expenses are associated with functions that must be performed regardless of the number of units of service being delivered, and other costs and expenses are incurred only when units of service are delivered. A departmental supervisor handles certain administrative duties regardless of patient levels, but the staffing of a second radiology technician on the afternoon shift is justified based on patient load requirements. (Staffing issues for smaller hospitals are discussed further in chapter 4.)

Allocated Expenses

Non–revenue-producing department costs distributed among revenue departments are called *allocated expenses.* Examples of non–revenue-producing departments include the business office, the medical record department, housekeeping, and administration. Allocated expenses include interest, depreciation, insurance, and hospitalwide management fees.

Controllable and Noncontrollable Expenses

Controllable expenses are expenses that fall under the control of a department manager and are charged directly to the department. Departmental salaries and supplies are examples of controllable expenses. *Noncontrollable expenses* are expenses that are not under the control of the manager, such as interest, depreciation, and insurance, and are charged indirectly to the department.

Direct and Indirect Expenses

Direct expenses are cost components for items specifically traceable to a unit of output and are assigned to a specific department. For example, X-ray film and lead jackets would be direct expenses for the radiology department. *Indirect expenses* are those labor, material, and equipment costs that are not specifically traceable to a specific unit of output. These expenses exist for the operation of the hospital as a whole and include cleaning supplies, pencils, ordering forms, and landscaping.

The Budget as a Monitoring Tool

A discussion of the budget as a monitoring tool should be prefaced by a few more definitions related to the budgetary process. A *fixed budget* is determined based on specific activity levels and does not vary with changes in volumes of activity. A *flexible budget* reflects expenses that vary with different levels of activity. One of the most important steps in the budgeting process is to report and analyze *variances*. A variance is the difference between actual results and budgeted figures. Attention to variances is the beginning of the continuous cost control improvement process.

The departmental budget summarizes a department's actual financial and statistical activity for a month and provides a total for the year compared to a flexible budget. The departmental budget is a communication tool between the CEO and the department manager. It also provides actual data for evaluating departmental performance and directing a manager's attention to potential problem areas. In addition, the actual financial and statistical data from the current year's budget are used to develop the following year's budget.

Components of the Departmental Budget

The departmental budget consists of a description column, as well as actual and budgeted values for the month and year to date, a discussion of variances, and an explanation of corrective action. Entries for a revenue-producing department under the description column (see figure 3-4) include units of service, revenues, direct expenses, operating profit, allocated expenses, and net profit contribution. Some of these entries (direct and allocated expenses) have already been defined, and the remaining terms are defined as follows:

- *Units of service:* These statistics measure inpatient and outpatient services, as well as any other patient services delivered by the hospital (that is, emergency, home health, respite care, and so forth).
- *Revenues:* Dollar amounts are awarded to units of service and expressed as revenue. These amounts are also, therefore, expressed in terms of inpatient and outpatient revenue, as well as any other appropriate revenue.
- *Operating profit:* This type of profit is the difference between revenue and direct expenses.
- *Net profit (contribution):* The difference between the operating profit and the allocated expenses is called the net profit.

In departmental budgets for non–revenue-producing departments, direct expenses are compared to total units of service and summarized on a per-unit basis. Monthly and year-to-date values are portrayed at actual, budgeted, and variance levels. The department manager may want to list values for the previous year, as well. A non–revenue-producing department should record explanations for variances and show what actions should be taken to resolve the problems.

Flexible Budgeting

Flexible budgeting uses a mathematical formula based on the fixed (or original) budget, as well as differences in revenue and expenses resulting from changes in the amount of units of service. Examples of items that are affected when flexing the budget include revenue, variable salaries, supplies, purchased services (departmental functions), and physician fees.

Figure 3-4. Sample Budget Reporting Format

Radiology

_____ (Month)

Description	Actual	Budget	Variance
Billable tests (units)			
Inpatient	950	1,520	−570
Outpatient	1,200	2,400	−1,200
Total billable tests	2,150	3,920	−1,770
Gross revenue			
Inpatient	$38,000	$60,800	−22,800
Outpatient	48,000	96,000	−48,000
Total gross revenue	$86,000	$156,800	−70,800
Expenses (direct)			
Salaries (variable)	$13,100	$13,720	+620
Salaries (fixed)	36,000	36,000	0
Total salaries	$49,100	$49,720	+620
Vacation/sick/holiday (variable)	3,928	3,978	+50
Supplies (variable)	17,050	17,248	+198
Medical fees (variable)	0	0	—
Other direct expenses	0	0	—
Total direct expenses	$70,078	$70,946	+868
Operating profit	15,922	85,854	−69,932
Allocated expenses	25,800	47,040	+21,240
Contribution	$−9,878	$38,814	−48,692

A department manager can develop a flexible monthly budget by using a form similar to the one shown in figure 3-4. The first step in developing a flexible monthly budget is to forecast utilization. For a radiology department, utilization can be expressed in billable tests, and can be retrieved from the hospital's prior year revenue and usage report, as illustrated in the budget column of the shaded section in figure 3-4.

Using the previous year's revenue by procedure and pay class (if available) and adjusting for inflation and third-party payment limits, the fiscal office of the hospital can develop a useful revenue-per-test ratio. For the example in figure 3-4, the revenue per test is $40.00. Revenue for the budget would then be shown in the gross revenue section of the budget column.

Once fixed and variable components have been determined, the direct expense components of the budget can be developed. All variable components should be based on forecasted units of service, trends from previous periods, and adjustments being made for the current year.

Once the direct expenses have been determined (expenses [direct] in figure 3-4), an operating profit can be quickly determined. After the allocation of expenses from non–revenue-producing departments, managers can arrive at their department's contribution. The basis for allocations may vary, depending on the department from which the allocation is being made (the amount of square feet the department takes up, the percentage of total operating costs, and so forth). The department head should focus on meeting or outperforming the budgeted amounts.

In flexible budgeting, it becomes important to forecast units of service, as well as resultant expenses and revenues based on historic trends, on a monthly basis. For example, some hospitals see significant differences in the numbers, complexity, and types of cases during the winter months as opposed to the summer months. As a result, it is important that each department consider seasonal trends, rather than simply forecasting each month by dividing the annual budget by 12. Of course, no matter how accurately a manager attempts to forecast each month, only through a flexible budget can one accurately gauge monthly performance.

Creation of a Flexible Budget

A fixed budget (the original budget) does not take into account that as units of service increase, so do revenue and variable costs. Therefore, variances between actual performance and the forecast performance can be deceiving in a fixed budget. To correct this phenomenon, a flexible budget sets targets for revenue and expenses that relate directly to the volume of service (units of service) experienced during a specific time.

Mathematical formulas are required to compute the flexible budget for each department. The following formulas are used to flex revenues and expenses:

$$\frac{\text{Fixed Revenue or Expense}}{\text{Fixed Units of Service}} = \frac{\text{Budgeted Amount}}{\text{per Unit of Service}}$$

$$\frac{\text{Budgeted Amount}}{\text{per Unit of Service}} \times \text{Actual Units of Service} = \frac{\text{Flexible}}{\text{Budget}}$$

When fixed budgets are compared to actual data, differences (variances) appear when there are changes to forecasted levels of activity. These fixed budget variances result in indications that could lead management to inappropriate areas for corrective action. Managers might miss the greatest opportunities for improvement.

Flexible budget comparisons enable management to focus on variances stemming from expenses that are under the control of a specific department manager. Variances will illustrate what expenses actually

were compared to what they should have been, relative to the actual
activity in that department. In expense analysis, those expenses labeled
as variable in the original budget should be flexed. Variances from the
flexed level of variable expenses usually present the best opportunities
to reduce costs. Flexible budget analysis should occur on a monthly basis,
with variances explained and corrective actions stated.

In figure 3-5, actual utilization is significantly less than forecasted
during the budget process. (Compare with figure 3-4.) Although utilization, revenue, and contribution amounts show negative variances in
figure 3-4, expenses display a positive variance. There is no indication
of which expenses management should consider reducing.

Figure 3-5. Sample Flexed Budget

Radiology

_____ (Month)

Description	Actual	Budget	Variance
Billable tests (units)			
Inpatient	950	—	—
Outpatient	1,200	—	—
Total billable tests	2,150	—	—
Gross revenue			
Inpatient	$38,000	—	—
Outpatient	48,000	—	—
Total gross revenue	$86,000	—	—
Expenses (direct)			
Salaries (variable)	$13,100	$ 7,525	−5,575
Salaries (fixed)	36,000	36,000	0
Total salaries	$49,100	$43,525	−5,575
Vacation/sick/holiday (variable)	3,928	3,482	−446
Supplies (variable)	17,050	9,460	−7,590
Medical fees (variable)	0	0	0
Other direct expenses	0	0	0
Total direct expenses	$70,078	$56,467	−13,611
Operating profit	15,922	29,533	
Allocated expenses	25,800	25,800	
Contribution	$−9,878	$ 3,733	

Explanation of Variances:
Salaries (variable):   We did not reduce worked hours as utilization dropped.

Corrective action: If utilization remains low this month, we will reduce one FTE on
third shift and one on second shift. We will also move one FTE
to stagger between the second and third shifts.

By flexing budgeted expenses to meet actual utilization, managers find it easier to visualize expense variances and opportunities for cost reduction. The variable budgeted expenses in figure 3-5 (that is, variable salaries, vacation/sick/holiday expenses, and supplies) have been altered to reflect actual utilization in the radiology department. The budgeted rate for variable salaries is $3.50 per radiology test (2,150 × $3.50 = $7,525 in variable salaries). Vacation, sick, and holiday expenses are budgeted at 8 percent of salaries ($43,525 × .08 = $3,482). Supplies are budgeted at $4.40 per test (2,150 × $4.40 = $9,460).

In figure 3-5, variable expenses in salaries and supplies have significantly higher variances than indicated by the fixed budget analysis in figure 3-4. This flexed approach to budgeting therefore directs management to investigate appropriate cost-containment opportunities.

The Effects of Variances on the Departmental Budget

If a department has a negative variance of $3.00, should there be an explanation? If managers investigated every variance, time-consuming and relatively meaningless reports would result, wasting the time of the reporter and the reviewer. To avoid this waste, minimum acceptable line-item variances between actual results and budgeted plans should be determined. Tolerance levels of 5 percent (year to date) and at least $1,500 on a monthly basis are good guidelines to consider. Each department's actual tolerance levels should be set by the hospital administrator.

Analysis of the Variances

As a variance becomes out of tolerance, the variance tends to be related solely to its effect on department profit contribution. Sometimes, however, variances showing that a department is over budget for revenues or under budget for expenses may not truly reflect "good" performance by the department. The following considerations might explain misleading variances:

- Significantly higher revenues (per unit of service) than budgeted plans could result from noncompetitive or uncollectible rate increases to offset higher-than-budgeted expenses.
- Higher expenses might be due to a failure to implement adequate cost-containment measures, even though the expenses are inside the budget limit.
- Significantly lower expenses than budgeted amounts in areas such as salaries could indicate an understaffing problem. Other quality-of-care issues could also arise from costs being below tolerance levels.

- The existing budget may have underestimated the department's ability to perform.

Through the use of analytical techniques, managers can determine why their department did not do as well as expected and formulate strategies to improve the situation. Most of this analysis involves the problem-solving steps (the creativity cycle) introduced in chapter 2. Interpretation of out-of-tolerance performance helps to identify departmental problems, determine the causes and effects of the problems, develop improved methods of service delivery, and monitor the success of solutions. Variance analysis also helps management to create more accurate budgets in the future.

Units of Revenue Variances

Figure 3-6 illustrates an instance when a laboratory department is experiencing revenue and utilization variances. The department is experiencing a favorable variance in utilization because the hospital performed more tests than budgeted. There could be several causes for these variances, including the initiation of new services that were not anticipated during the budgeting process or higher inpatient traffic resulting from a recently recruited internal medicine physician.

The laboratory department displays an unfavorable variance, however, in revenue performance. This variance is of additional concern considering that department utilization is reported to be high. As a result, the department also demonstrates an unfavorable variance in revenue per unit. The following might be possible reasons for these unfavorable variances:

- A rate increase was not implemented as budgeted.
- The hospital has been experiencing a higher level of lost charges.
- There has been a change in the types of patients being treated, resulting in a lower severity of illness and the ordering of less-costly tests.
- Physicians have been performing more of the expensive laboratory services in their offices.
- The hospital has begun a new service or has purchased new equipment that generates a lower revenue per unit of service.

The analysis of revenue and usage behavior helps managers understand cost behavior. If there is a lost charge problem, delivery-of-service costs may be higher than those being reported. If patients visiting the hospital have a lower-than-normal severity of illness, the unit cost of care should not be as high.

Figure 3-6. Sample Variances for a Laboratory Department

	Actual	Budget	Variance	Last Year
Billable tests	35,074	28,500	6,574	27,900
Revenue	$623,000	$705,000	$−82,000	$580,000
Revenue/unit	17.76	24.74	−12.47	20.79

Expense Variances

The largest dollar cost savings typically fall into the payroll-related (salary and wages, vacation/sick/holiday) expense areas. Supplies are also an area needing specific attention when variances are identified. (Methods to control payroll and supply costs are discussed at length in chapters 4 and 5.) All of these areas, however, are directly affected by the actions of the medical staff (as discussed in chapter 6). A review of budget variances becomes a process of exploring causes and effects.

Salaries and Wages

Salaries and wages are the first expense item on which to focus attention, for obvious reasons. Salaries and wages represent the single largest expense item in a budget, and they directly affect other expense areas such as education and training expenses, administrative expenses, and other payroll expenses (that is, health benefits; life insurance; accrued sick, vacation, and holiday time; and the employer's share of federal, state, and local taxes). Although it is a natural tendency to address payroll expenses when they are over budget, it is equally important to pay close attention when they are under budget. Often, understaffing problems that surface today can lead to quality problems tomorrow. Consequently, it is in the manager's best interest to closely monitor payroll expenses.

The following are some reasons why payroll expenses may be out of tolerance (positively or negatively):

- Overtime, call-back, and standby pay
- More or fewer employees on hand
- A different mix of employees
- Actual pay rates different from budgeted pay rates

Determining the cause or combination of causes for out-of-tolerance salary expenses requires analysis of actual expenses versus budgeted expenses, as well as an analysis of past expense trends. The best ratios to use for this analysis are the average hourly pay rate and hours worked per various units of measure (that is, worked hours per case weight-adjusted stay, per billable test, per observation hour, per patient day, per square foot maintained, per pounds of laundry, per meals served, and so forth).

For example, a radiology department shows that more hours than usual are being worked per test. The following explanations might surface:

- *More time-consuming tests are being performed.* If this possibility is suggested, verification may come from reviewing revenue and usage reports. An important factor in determining a price for a specific procedure is the amount of time it takes to complete it (although some might argue that price determination depends more on how many procedures are performed for patients with charge-based paying insurance coverage and what the payer determines to be the allowable charge). There would be three ways to alleviate the variance: the budget could be adjusted to reflect higher revenue per test for the same period of time; the budgeted hours per test could be adjusted; or a lower-cost alternative to the tests being performed could be suggested.
- *Each employee is experiencing lower productivity.* Perhaps the volume of tests performed was not adequate to achieve anticipated economies of scale. It may make sense to review the time of day tests are being run to determine more efficient methods of staffing and scheduling elective procedures. Productivity might also appear to be lower because of the following:
  - Fewer tests are being performed by outside services.
  - Established testing standards are not realistic.
  - Equipment is not performing well, requiring significant retakes.

Vacation/Sick Time/Holiday

Vacations, sick time, and holidays are components of another expense area to consider when budget variances appear. Dollars for this expense are recorded in the month they are paid. If there are three payrolls paid in one month (as occasionally happens in a 31-day month), this expense will appear to be high. When this expense appears high, the year-to-date expense should be examined to determine whether problems exist. If vacation/sick time/holiday expense still appears to be high, the following questions should be asked:

- Were more people taking sick days this year than last year?
- Did employees use more vacation time during the winter holiday season this year than last year?

- Did employees use more vacation days than time off without pay to meet reduced staffing needs?

Supplies

A review of ratios, along with data from the hospital's purchase records, is usually required to analyze supply expense variances. Supply expenses are usually the most controllable expense item in the budget after payroll-related expenses. Although the materials manager is usually assumed to control these expenses, others in the hospital (such as department personnel and physicians) can significantly affect supply expenses through their ordering habits. Similar to vacation/sick time/holiday expenses, the year-to-date variance in supply expenses becomes more important than the month-by-month reported variance.

As variances in supply expenses are investigated, the hospital's purchase journal should be reviewed to answer the following questions:

- What has been done with the supplies expensed from the purchase journal? Have they been used or are they still on the inventory shelf? Is the last in−first out (LIFO) or the first in−first out (FIFO) method of accounting being used to account for the expense? The answers to these questions help determine whether, through appropriate inventory control, supply costs will decrease in the future.
- Are supplies being wasted, stolen, or lost? Often the charging system is a good place to begin finding answers to this question. By determining who is the last accountable agent in the supply-issuing process, a manager may pinpoint the locations and causes of a variance.
- Was there previously a supply backlog that is now being processed?
- Have the unit purchase costs increased? Invoice prices should be compared to order prices and purchasing contracts to ensure that the predetermined prices are being honored by hospital vendors. If prices are higher but within the terms of hospital agreements, then the budget may need to be adjusted (assuming the hospital cannot renegotiate purchasing contracts or find less-costly alternatives).
- Is the hospital getting what it is paying for? Are receipt inspections occurring upon delivery, and are records of these inspections on file and checked by the accounts payable section prior to payment?

The budgeting process also helps the hospital make critical decisions beyond the scope of the operating budget itself. For example, the hospital may determine that the labor variance in radiology is, in part, being caused by a defective radiographic/fluoroscopic (R/F) table. The amount of retakes, for instance, may require more work hours per billable test, as well as a higher variable cost for film. Replacement of the R/F table may significantly reduce both payroll and supply expenses. As these issues present themselves, the hospital must turn to capital planning and budgeting.

Capital Planning and Budgeting

The continual provision of health care services requires a significant investment in capital for any hospital. For smaller hospitals, capital investment is a critical decision process because funds and access to financing are so limited. Because of limited funds and access to financing, many smaller hospitals will close their doors over the next 10 years. Those smaller hospitals that survive will have successfully carried out well-developed capital plans.

Strategic and Financial Management

Like the operational budget, the capital budget must be linked to the hospital's strategic plan. The capital budget must also be consistent with the hospital's mission and overall direction as established by the trustees, management, and medical staff. A strategic plan that complements the hospital's mission and direction will best meet the community's health care needs.

Managing the financial assets used to acquire capital is a significant challenge. Although this responsibility rests with the hospital administrator, the authority to perform this function in a smaller hospital may be delegated to its chief financial officer (when there is one). Management faces several limitations as it pursues its capital plan. Hospital administrators must acquire financial resources to fund current operations, as well as resources for their hospital's current and future capital requirements. Equally challenging are decisions to invest in existing or new business lines. Important to this decision is input from the hospital's medical staff. The physicians, after all, are the individuals who significantly control the care of patients. They can provide vital information as to which business lines are needed and worthy of investigation.

The ultimate source of capital financing is income derived from hospital operations. Income from operations either directly funds capital acquisition or is used to pay the debt service. Most financial institutions require hospitals to maintain certain key ratios in their loan covenants that are at least partially based on income from operations. Some even argue that when a hospital's capital source is a local tax referendum, it is management's responsibility to demonstrate fiscal responsibility to generate a profit so that alternative funding sources can be used in the future.

Key Elements in Capital Planning

There are three key elements to capital planning. First, the current capital budget is the planning and controlling mechanism for the capital expenditures and for financing those expenditures. The capital budget should be included in the hospital's overall budget. The capital budget consists of the following:

- Current expenditures for new equipment
- Routine maintenance and improvement of the physical plant
- Equipment repair and replacement
- The current portion of any long-term project

Second, the capital plan is typically a three-to-five-year master plan for current and long-term capital expenditures. The capital plan is management's tool for linking the hospital's strategic goals to a set of planned capital expenditures. Using strategic and financial criteria, management can set its priorities for expenditures. The capital plan should also include potential sources of funds for these outlays, as well as the hospital's approach to obtaining these funds. As the hospital's strategic goals shift, the capital plan must be revised along with the capital budget.

The third element of capital planning consists of the capital structure being developed as a result of the hospital's implemented capital plan. The capital structure consists of the hospital's mix of debt and owner-invested funds. Also included in the structure are the rights and responsibilities assigned to certain owner-invested funds. The capital structure will influence how the hospital approaches capital markets in the future. In other words, the capital structure will affect capital planning.

Capital Expenditures

The capital budget process is the final step in the planning and evaluation of proposals for investments in property, facilities, and equipment. Various distinct but related steps are taken in analyzing and deciding among various expenditures. By following these steps, management stands a better chance of selecting the right expenditures, as well as obtaining the governing board's approval.

Koval and Mikhail, contributors to the recent book *Hospital Capital Formation: Strategies and Tactics for the 1990s,* recommend that the hospital take seven steps in the capital selection process. These steps are listed and explained in figure 3-7.

Murphy's law decrees that every project will take twice as long, be twice as expensive, and prove half as effective as originally expected. Often there can be more types of costs than originally anticipated. To

Figure 3-7.   The Capital Budget Process

Step 1: Develop guidelines.

- A timetable is set for identifying expenditures, developing the budget, and submitting the budget for approval.
- Preliminary spending levels are determined.
- The information necessary to make the decisions is specified.

Step 2: Identify specific projects.

- A preliminary cost–benefit analysis is developed for each project.
- Projects are evaluated and ranked.
- Management identifies the effects these project decisions will have on hospital and department plans.

Step 3: Total and review capital requests.

- Capital requests are compared to available funds and for appropriateness to the strategic plan.
- Each request is ranked and prioritized.

Step 4: Determine final capital budget.

- Total expenditure limits are set.
- Final lists of projects are determined.
- Contingency funds are set aside.

Step 5: Capital budget is approved by board.

Step 6: Individual projects are submitted to board for approval or commitment.

- Final cost–benefit analysis or feasibility studies are completed.
- Preliminary capital cost estimates are set.
- Method and sources of financing are identified.
- Individual project packages are submitted to the board complete with above information and a detailed implementation plan.

Step 7: Monitor performance of approved projects.

- Progress reports are made according to implementation plans.
- A postcompletion audit is performed.

Adapted from A. F. Koval and O. I. Mikhail, Identifying Capital Needs. In: A. T. Solovy, ed., *Hospital Capital Formation: Strategies and Tactics for the 1990s* (Chicago: American Hospital Publishing, 1991), p. 25.

help disprove Murphy's law, Koval and Mikhail again recommend that the hospital use the list of costs found in figure 3-8 in feasibility studies or cost–benefit analyses.

Figure 3-8. Capital Budget Checklist

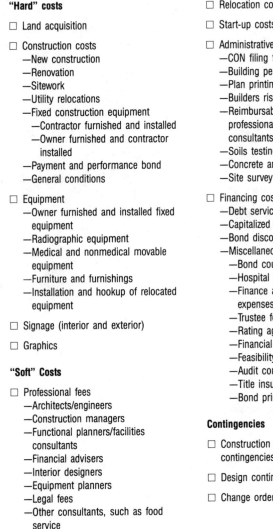

"Hard" costs

☐ Land acquisition

☐ Construction costs
—New construction
—Renovation
—Sitework
—Utility relocations
—Fixed construction equipment
  —Contractor furnished and installed
  —Owner furnished and contractor installed
—Payment and performance bond
—General conditions

☐ Equipment
—Owner furnished and installed fixed equipment
—Radiographic equipment
—Medical and nonmedical movable equipment
—Furniture and furnishings
—Installation and hookup of relocated equipment

☐ Signage (interior and exterior)

☐ Graphics

"Soft" Costs

☐ Professional fees
—Architects/engineers
—Construction managers
—Functional planners/facilities consultants
—Financial advisers
—Interior designers
—Equipment planners
—Legal fees
—Other consultants, such as food service

☐ Relocation costs

☐ Start-up costs

☐ Administrative expenses
—CON filing fee
—Building permit fees
—Plan printing
—Builders risk insurance premiums
—Reimbursable expenses of professionals (that is, architects, consultants)
—Soils testing and borings
—Concrete and steel testing
—Site survey

☐ Financing costs
—Debt service reserve fund
—Capitalized interest
—Bond discount or placement fee
—Miscellaneous financing expenses
  —Bond counsel
  —Hospital legal counsel
  —Finance authority fee and expenses
  —Trustee fee
  —Rating agencies
  —Financial adviser
  —Feasibility study
  —Audit comfort
  —Title insurance premium
  —Bond printing

Contingencies

☐ Construction cost estimating contingencies

☐ Design contingencies

☐ Change orders

Adapted from A. F. Koval and O. I. Mikhail, Identifying Capital Needs. In: A. T. Solovy, ed., *Hospital Capital Formation: Strategies and Tactics for the 1990s* (Chicago: American Hospital Publishing, 1991), p. 35.

Conclusion

Both operational budgets and capital budgets serve as tools for the smaller hospital's management and board of trustees to plan, monitor, and evaluate the hospital's financial performance. As a result of the effective use of budgets and budgeting techniques, a hospital can make better-informed decisions concerning its future. Only with a well-developed budget can a hospital predict the results of proposed operating alternatives with some level of confidence. As hospital management becomes more skilled at identifying variances from established standards and testing alternative approaches, some real improvements will be made in service efficiency.

Bibliography

Finkler, S. A. *The Complete Guide to Finance and Accounting for Nonfinancial Managers.* Englewood Cliffs, NJ: Prentice-Hall, 1983.

Nackel, J. G., Kis, G. M., and Feneroli, P. J. *Cost Management for Hospitals.* Rockville, MD: Aspen Publishers, 1987.

Solovy, A. T., editor. *Hospital Capital Formation: Strategies and Tactics for the 1990s.* Chicago: American Hospital Publishing, 1991.

Chapter 4

Controlling Labor Costs

Most smaller hospitals face a fierce challenge in controlling labor costs. The problem of attracting skilled nursing and allied health professionals, at a time when those skills are in short supply, makes close control of labor utilization a delicate issue. But no area is more important to cost control. Labor costs are the single largest component of health care operating costs. In a hospital at risk of failure, focusing on control over staffing often presents the best opportunity for cost reduction and more appropriate use of scarce labor skills.

Among the smaller hospitals that closed during the early years of the prospective payment system, many were experiencing relatively high staffing levels (in excess of 4.5 full-time equivalents [FTEs] per adjusted patient day).[1] Successful smaller hospitals usually operated at much lower staffing levels (between 3.0 and 3.5 FTEs per adjusted patient day). The smaller hospitals that were failing either did not know which areas to reduce or did not act on the areas identified as problems.[2]

The Philosophy of Productivity

There are two ways of looking at the productivity problem. In exploring labor issues, the hospital's dilemma is whether to reduce the number of people served or to increase the level of business. In resolving this dilemma, it is important to remember that productivity requires obtaining optimal results from available resources. These results may be realized through reduced operating costs, increased productivity, and a more efficient team accomplishing management's goals.

Productivity has two sides: reducing the amount of staff where there are too many workers and placing staff in areas where there are too few workers or none at all. Unfortunately, some failing hospitals have done a very good job of the former but have neglected the latter. Successful productivity involves closely monitoring the hospital's investment in people and developing new methods and services as needed. When financially draining and overstaffed hospital departments keep doing the same old tasks the same old way, improving productivity is impossible. Productivity is replaced by staff reductions and eventual discontinuations of services.

A productivity system helps administrators determine whether and how they can effectively use hospital resources. Accurate and achievable productivity standards can only be developed through direct observation of and discussions with the managers and employees of each department. Administrators cannot merely assume that departmental standards are interchangeable among different hospitals.

Typically, a productivity monitoring system can improve productivity by a reasonable amount (from 10 to 30 percent) without disturbing employees' work patterns. The improved productivity is achieved through the following innovations:

- Instituting proper staffing levels
- Reducing the amount of idle time
- Improving work methods
- Eliminating "personal" time
- Controlling work flow
- Improving the quality of supervision
- Teaching personnel to supervise themselves

The development of a productivity monitoring system requires the identification of performance standards for each hospital department. Such standards enable the hospital to identify areas needing improved work flows. Performance standards also identify where work is being duplicated and where unnecessary work has been assigned to staff.

The Productivity Monitoring System

A way to monitor labor costs on a continuing basis is to use a productivity monitoring system. Productivity monitoring systems can be elaborate computer-driven data systems, or they can be as simple as a handwritten form. A performance standard, or index, is developed for each area or department to be evaluated. This standard is based on a unit of measure, such as patient days, billable tests, visits, square feet, and so forth. Managers should evaluate variances (over and under) from performance standards and determine appropriate corrective actions.

Critical Components of Productivity

It is important that managers understand the different types of time units found in a productivity monitoring system and how these time units should be used. The time units evaluated in a productivity monitoring system are the worked hours for the period being evaluated. Time-unit reports are completed either every pay period (the easiest method because the worked hours can be extracted from payroll reports) or every month (to coincide with financial reports).

Many larger hospitals develop performance standards based only on variable hours of staffing. Unlike larger hospitals, smaller hospitals must give an appropriate value for constant hours as well. Standards in smaller hospitals are represented as worked hours and are given constant, variable, and minimum considerations.

Constant hours are activities not directly related to departmental units of service, such as administrative support, orientation programs, educational inservices, and other "nonproductive" time. One of the driving factors in determining constant hours is the number of hours per day a department remains open, regardless of patient load. As utilization changes, the constant hour standard for the department remains the same.

Variable hours are worked hours allowed per unit of service. As utilization increases, the variable hour standard increases. As utilization decreases, the variable hour standard decreases. In developing the department standard, the variable hour standard is added to the constant hour standard. If there is no utilization during the evaluated period, no variable hours would be added to the constant hour component of the standard.

Examples of variable hours on a departmental basis are shown in figure 4-1. The variable staffing for medical/surgical nursing is increased by 6 hours for each medical/surgical patient day during a two-week pay period. To determine total medical/surgical nursing hours for a period, the variable hours are multiplied by the number of medical/surgical patient days reported for that period and then added to the constant hour standard. If the hospital reported 100 patient days for a pay period, then the constant hours (372 hours) plus the variable hours (6 hours multiplied by 100 patient days, or 600 hours) would equal 972 hours.

Minimum hours are hours allowed when constant and variable hours combined do not reach a predetermined level needed to meet safety requirements. In the medical/surgical example described in the preceding paragraph, the calculated value for constant and variable hours (972 hours) is less than the established minimum hour standard (1,008 hours) for the department. Therefore the standard in this example would be 1,008 hours. Such standards are developed for each hospital department and are driven by the units of service associated with each department. For each department, the standard hours are compared to the actual worked hours to determine a ratio, or performance index, upon which to base appropriate action.

Figure 4-1. Examples of Labor Standards for Smaller Hospitals

Department	Unit of Measure	Standard (Worked) Hours per 14-Day Period		
		Constant	Variable	Minimum
Nursing				
Administration	Constant	80	—	—
Med/Surg	Med/Surg patient days	372	6	1,008
ICU	ICU patient days	118	12	336
OB/Gyn	Deliveries		9	336
	OB patient days		4.5	—
	Nursery days		24<14 days	—
			12>14 days	—
OR/Recovery	Minutes	80	0.08	240
Emergency	ER visits	118	1.0	336
Pharmacy	Pharmacy units	40	1.0	240
Laboratory	Billable tests	96	0.2	240
Respiratory	RVUs therapy	96	0.25	224
EKGs	EKG tests	10	0.25	—
Radiology	Billable tests	96	0.6	240
Dietary	Total meals	—	0.29	560
Medical records	Discharges	80	2.0	240
	OP surgeries	—	1.0	—
	ER/OP visits	—	0.1	—
Maintenance	Patient days	80	0.05	80
Housekeeping	Patient days	80	0.17	716
Business office	Admissions	500	2.0	—
	ER/OP visits	—	0.5	—
Administration	Constant	320	—	—

Development of Labor Standards

Many managers do not like the idea of setting labor standards. They do not enjoy devising rules that become the basis for measuring staff performance. However, meeting departmental labor standards can be a source of personal, departmental, and hospitalwide pride.

There are three ways to determine hospital labor standards. The estimated standard approach is the simplest method and entails the lowest cost. These standards are established by dividing 12 months of worked departmental hours by the number of units of measure that each department uses. The resulting standard is the historical number of units worked per hour.

Another method of determining hospital labor standards is to use engineered standards. Engineered standards are developed by first identifying all the units of work in a department. Then the time required to complete each unit is determined, along with the frequency with which each task is performed.

A third way to determine labor standards is to use time-value units (TVUs). Time-value units are predetermined values assigned to each chargeable procedure, and they represent the average time it takes a qualified technician to perform a procedure in an appropriate and professional manner. These units are usually considered "industry-accepted" standards that can then be adjusted for local peculiarities. The national professional organization for each technical specialty typically develops these standards.

Every hospital has unique conditions that must be considered when standards are being developed. Therefore, standards cannot be developed for one hospital and then automatically applied to another hospital. In developing hospital labor standards, the department manager or an outside party such as a consultant should survey each department. The surveyor should:

- Measure daily work loads for both clinical and administrative areas
- Identify, in detail, all department-billable activities
- Specify frequency and duration of educational programs, supervisory responsibilities, and other activities unaffected by fluctuations in the volume of departmental units of measure
- Identify any significant barriers or problems stemming from the physical plant, equipment, medical staff relations, and so forth

After hospital departmental surveys have been completed, four elements determine the standard for each department: units of service, variable hours, constant hours, and minimum hours. An example set of standards for a 75-bed hospital is illustrated in figure 4-1. And although examples are helpful, every hospital must develop its own standards based on these four elements. Some compromises will also be necessary to achieve departmental agreement on standards staff feels to be achievable.

Recognizing the Difference between Constant and Minimum Hours

Smaller hospitals with high salary costs typically overcompensate the constant (or fixed) portion of staffing budgets. One approach is to maintain constant staffing at a level allowing the hospital to adequately staff for peak patient loads. This philosophy emphasizes retainment of skilled labor and acknowledges that smaller hospitals' patient volumes can fluctuate dramatically over a short period of time. As a result, hospitals using this philosophy assign a high constant component, leading to little or no change in worked hours as units of service change.

In a medical/surgical nursing department, for example, staffing with this approach may lead to the staffing pattern illustrated in figure 4-2. The staffing does not reflect adjustment based on varying units of service; rather, staffing adjustments are based on the availability of nurses. It may be surprising to note that staffing is higher for the lowest patient period (210 patient days) than for the period with the highest patient load (460 patient days). The worked-hour fluctuations reflected in figure 4-2 are the result of employees taking vacation days and sick days. Hospitals that show a constant staffing pattern are likely to supplement staff with temporary agency nurses.

Another cause for higher-than-necessary staffing is a misunderstanding of the difference between constant and minimum staffing. A hospital may mistakenly increase its labor standards by adding the variable component for all units of service to the established minimum amount, instead of to the constant amount. In a smaller hospital, where units of service are sometimes very low, the minimum staffing standard will occasionally be utilized. However, it is important to remember that minimum hours are a factor in the development of standards only when units of service do not drive staffing levels to minimum amounts dictated by hospital policy and state licensing and certification requirements.

Determining the Constant Amount

Determining each department's hourly standard requires an understanding of how the department operates. To help understand a department's operation, the following questions should be asked:

- How many hours is the department open daily?
- Is an administrative person needed? If so, for how many hours daily?
- How much time does the supervisor spend performing daily administrative functions, regardless of patient levels?

Once the amount of departmental activity in these areas is determined, the constant component of the standard can be developed by computing the activity amount for the period being evaluated. For example, in figure 4-1 the constant for a 14-day pay period on the medical/surgical floor, 372 hours, represents the worked hours of a ward clerk on the 7 to 3 and 3 to 11 shifts each day, as well as four hours per shift of the floor supervisor's non–patient care time. This constant would be computed as follows:

Ward clerk = 14 (days) × 8 (hours) × 2 (shifts) = 224 hours

Supervisor = 14 (days) × 4 (hours) × 3 (shifts) = 168 hours

Total constant hours = 392 hours

Determining the Variable Amount

A variable amount is driven by the actual units of service performed. A single value is established to represent the time required to produce an amount of departmental service in a particular period of time. The variable amount for medical/surgical nursing (as shown in figure 4-1) is 6 hours of nursing care per patient day. If the hospital had a patient census of 280 patient days for the 14-day period (that is, an average daily census of 20), the variable medical/surgical nursing component for that period would be:

6 (hours) × 280 (patient days) = 1,680 worked hours

Determining the Minimum Amount

Minimum amounts of staffing are based on hospital and state-driven requirements. For the medical/surgical nursing example in figure 4-2, the amount might be a minimum of three full-time equivalents (FTEs) in the hospital at all times. If, during any pay period, the constant amount plus the variable amount is less than the identified minimum amount, then staffing for that period would equal the minimum amount.

Figure 4-2. Example of Highly Constant Staffing in One Smaller Hospital

Patient Days (Medical/Surgical) per Pay Period	Worked Hours per Pay Period
210	2,745
221	2,735
245	2,685
318	2,742
355	2,785
325	2,770
375	2,765
460	2,735

Therefore, again using the preceding example, the total medical/ surgical nursing staffing standard for a 14-day period can be calculated by following these steps:

Constant + Variable   = Total
392 hours + 1,680 hours = 2,072 hours
Minimum staffing = 3 (FTEs) × 24 (hours) × 14 (days)
                 = 1,008 hours

Because the constant plus variable amount (2,072 hours) is greater than the minimum amount (1,008 hours), the staffing standard would be 2,072 hours for that time period.

If the average daily census had only been 5 patients (70 patient days), the constant plus variable amount would have been 812 hours (392 hours + 420 hours). In this case, the standard for the period would have been the 1,008-hour minimum amount.

Evaluation of Performance

Although numbers never tell the whole story, a quantitative measure for gauging departmental performance is a good place to begin evaluation. The first step in evaluating performance is calculating the department's performance indexes. Expressed as a percentage of standard performance, the index shows the degree to which the department is operating productively.

For the staffing analysis shown in figure 4-3, the performance indexes are calculated by dividing the standard level of hours for the department

Figure 4-3. Sample Calculations of Performance Indexes

Department	Standard	Actual	Performance Index
Nursing	1,536	1,843	0.83
Laboratory	452	416	1.08
Radiology	360	270	1.33
Pharmacy	151	154	0.98
Respiratory	125	99	1.26
Medical records	304	242	1.26
Business office	823	476	1.73
Dietary	755	714	1.06
Housekeeping	382	370	1.03
Maintenance	119	119	1.00
Purchasing	80	80	1.00
Administration	320	320	1.00
Total	5,407	5,103	1.06

by the actual hours worked during a specific time period. For example, if the standard hours in nursing were 1,536 hours and the actual worked nursing hours were 1,843, then the performance index for that department would be 83.3 percent of standard. If a performance index shows a variance of more than 10 percent from the standard, then the department head should investigate and report the reason for the variance to administration.

If the number of hours actually worked is lower than the standard, then the performance index will be greater than 1.00. In keeping with the preceding example, if the actual worked hours were only 1,200, then the performance index for the 1,536-hour standard would be 1.28. Although the administration may want to celebrate when a department reports such a performance index, a value over 1.10 should also be investigated and reported. Understaffing can lead to even larger problems than overstaffing.

A detailed staffing analysis is illustrated in figure 4-4. In this analysis, overtime recorded during the pay period is listed so that management can begin to identify potential problems beyond the staffing performance index. In this example, the hospital's medical/surgical nursing staff is being cross-utilized in the nursery, intensive care unit (ICU), and emergency departments. As a result, medical/surgical nursing appears to be overstaffed, and other nursing service areas appear to be understaffed. This report also indicates the high level of overtime under medical/surgical nursing, where almost two FTEs (158 hours) were paid at time and a half. Some further explanation is needed. The nursery standard in figure 4-4 shows the minimum standard due to low volume (15 nursery patient days) during the pay period.

Figure 4-5 represents a better reflection of hospital staffing. In that figure, the effect of the cross-training and sharing of staff is clearer. Staffing performance in the nursing departments with and without ambulance staffing is compared.

The Cross-Training of Staff

The only way for a hospital to fully utilize staff is by training them to perform several different functions. For example, a smaller hospital may not have the labor resources to be able to employ nurses who only work in the intensive care unit, or only in surgery, or only on medical/surgical floors. Successful hospitals cross-utilize staff to the fullest extent possible.

Management is usually going to experience some level of resistance to staff-sharing initiatives. Often, hospital managers will have already attempted to cross-train employees and feel they have tried every possible staffing combination. In other cases, the idea is so foreign to hospital staff that they cannot believe the concept could work.

Figure 4-4.   Sample Staffing Analysis

General Hospital Labor Performance Report **Pay Period Ending 8/17/93**						
Department	**Unit of Measure**	**Volume**	**Standard**	**Worked Hours**	**Overtime**	**Performance Index**
Nursing administration	Total patient days	384	80	80	0	1.00
Medical/surgical	M/S and OB days	380	2,160	2,496	158	0.81
Intensive care unit	Intensive care unit days	4	96	48	3	1.88
Labor room	Deliveries	5	45	45	0	1.00
Nursery	Nursery patient days	15	336	80	18	3.43
OR/recovery room	Minutes	60	4	4	0	1.00
Emergency	ER visits	266	266	216	12	1.17
Pharmacy	Pharmacy units	71	151	154	4	0.96
Laboratory	Billable tests	1,703	452	416	32	1.01
Respiratory	RVUs	143	96	70	59	0.74
EKG/EEG	EKG/EEG tests	118	29	29	0	1.00
Radiology	Billable tests	441	360	270	51	1.12
Medical records	Discharges	106	304	242	9	1.21
	OP surgery	1	—	—	—	—
	ER/OP visits	916	—	—	—	—
Dietary	Total meals	2,816	755	717	9	1.04
Housekeeping/ laundry	Square feet	26.6	382	370	25	0.97
	Total patient days	384	—	—	—	—
Maintenance	Square feet	26.6	119	119	0	1.00
Administration	Total patient days	384	240	233	1	1.03
Utilization review	Total patient days	384	80	80	0	1.00
Data processing	Total patient days	384	141	141	2	0.99
Business office	IP/OP registration	1,022	823	476	21	1.66
Accounting	Total patient days	384	80	80	0	1.00
Purchasing	Total patient days	384	160	171	0	0.94
Subtotal	—	—	7,159	6,537	404	1.03
Ambulance	Trips	60	448	661	10	0.67
Total	—	—	7,607	7,198	414	1.00

Figure 4-5. Summary Labor Performance Report

	Combined Standard	Total Worked Hours	Total Overtime	Combined Performance Index
Nursing departments (without ambulance)	2,987	2,969	191	0.95
Nursing departments (with ambulance)	3,435	3,630	201	0.90
Ancillary departments	1,088	939	146	1.00
Support departments	1,560	1,448	43	1.05
Administration/ fiscal services	1,524	1,181	24	1.26
Total	7,607	7,198	414	1.00

Guidelines for Resource Sharing

Through a deliberate staff analysis, the hospital can overcome some obstacles to resource sharing. The following are some steps that can lead to a better use of available staff:

- Determine true resource requirements based on work-load fluctuations.
- Identify appropriate staff to shift from a home department to an area of need.
- Accurately calculate and report productivity changes resulting from resource sharing.
- Assign jobs within the capabilities of workers, and adequately train staff in the performance of new functions.
- Provide appropriate financial incentives, as needed.
- Make sure everyone involved in the resource-sharing process clearly understands the hospital's objectives and why they are important.

Figure 4-6 illustrates general guidelines for how a hospital might share its nurses, provided there are no restrictions on such a practice, such as those imposed by unions. Ideally, hospital departments will list as many positive answers as possible. The chart should be read across to determine which recipient departments could effectively utilize nurses from a donor department. For example, available nurses from the emergency department (ED) could temporarily work in surgery (OR), intensive care (ICU), medical/surgical nursing (medical/surgical), or the obstetrics wing (OB), but not in the nursing home or home health service.

Figure 4-6. Sample Resource-Sharing Guidelines (Nursing)

Donors	ED	OR	ICU	Medical/ surgical	OB	Nursing Home	Home Health
				Recipients			
ED	—	Yes	Yes	Yes	Yes	No	No
OR	Yes	—	Yes	Yes	Yes	Yes	No
ICU	Yes	No	—	Yes	No	Yes	Yes
Medical/surgical	No	No	Yes	—	Yes	Yes	Yes
OB	No	Yes	Yes	Yes	—	Yes	Yes
Nursing home	No	No	No	Yes	No	—	Yes
Home health	No	No	No	Yes	No	Yes	—

Alternatively, by reading down a column, a manager can determine where a recipient department could look within the organization to find nursing staff donors. An OR manager needing supplemental staff should first look to the ED or OB for available staff. Using these guidelines as a springboard, along with the creativity cycle discussed in chapter 2, hospitals can explore their own resource-sharing potential.

Effective staff sharing requires more than a willingness to float resources during volume shifts. Policies must be developed so that everyone understands when and how shared staff will shift and to whom shared staff will report. Nurse managers must closely scrutinize assignments to ensure that proper care guidelines are followed.

Case Study

When a particular CEO of a county hospital in Georgia is asked about resource sharing, he admits that his hospital began the practice as a matter of survival. The county hospital has survived quite well, with plentiful cash reserves and a continuously profitable operation on an average daily census of 30 patients (70 percent Medicare and Medicaid).

The hospital had been faced with a common smaller hospital productivity problem—operating with too few nurses to utilize traditional staffing methods. The hospital had only 12 registered nurses to staff all emergency, medical/surgical, intensive care, and obstetrics services. Through several meetings and experiments, hospital staff and management developed the most comprehensive cross-sharing staffing plan possible.

The hospital typically operated below 3.5 FTEs per adjusted patient day, a figure that includes the hospital's ambulance service and regional renal dialysis center. For a given pay period, the hospital averaged 26.6

patients per day (373 patient visits over 14 days), and staffed all areas of the hospital with 102 FTEs. When it is considered that outpatient revenue represented 30 percent of total revenue at that time, the overall staffing for an adjusted average census of 34.6 days was 2.95 FTEs per adjusted patient day.

The hospital was able to maintain these impressive ratios through extensive cross-training of staff. The ED now provides physician-staffed service 24 hours per day, with medical/surgical, OB, and OR nurses cross-trained to work there as well. The OR staff consists of one RN supervisor and an additional RN who only works three days per week. One of these two nurses covers the ED or OB when no surgeries are being performed. The OR staff is also cross-trained to perform sterile processing. The nurse supervisor on the medical/surgical 7-to-3 shift serves as the emergency department nurse when the operating room staff is unavailable.

The respiratory department uses three FTEs from 6:00 a.m. to 4:30 p.m. and utilizes a call-back system for the remaining hours. The respiratory staff also works as pharmacy aides, nurses' aides, and as members of the ambulance crew when not performing respiratory, pulmonary, electroencephalography, and electrocardiography functions. All members of the pharmacy staff (two full-time pharmacists, two full-time technicians, and one part-time technician) also work on the respiratory or ambulance staff when needed.

Granted, this county hospital may have implemented resource sharing out of necessity, but it is extremely important for every hospital to implement this practice. If a hospital's clinical, financial, and administrative functions can be executed in the most resource-conservative fashion, then other resources can be focused on developing new hospital programs, training staff, educating the community, and planning how health care will be provided in the future.

Almost 15 years ago, the county hospital in this case study developed a freestanding renal dialysis center, which now serves a major portion of rural southeast Georgia. The hospital has also pioneered the creation of a health care cooperative consisting of 16 hospitals. The county hospital consistently reports approximately $500,000 revenue in excess of expenses. When tribute is paid for the hospital's success, its CEO modestly claims, "I really have had very little to do with it." The CEO has attained his objectives with and through the voluntary cooperation and efforts of others, making this county hospital an exemplary model of resource sharing.

Staffing and Scheduling

Hospital staffing and scheduling are handled at the department level. Department heads, especially new ones, often have no significant training in staffing dynamics and tend to view the staffing function as the mere filling of vacancies. However, the function of staffing involves a great deal more, including forecasting long-term personnel needs, planning for orientation and training, implementing job rotations, and instituting interdepartmental sharing. Prior to filling any vacancy, department heads should briefly evaluate their staffing situations, asking the following questions:

- Is the vacant job's function still necessary?
- Could existing staff perform the job's tasks?
- Are skills required for the vacant job missing among the staff?
- If the department added a new member, what kind of person would contribute the most to team effectiveness?
- Could the vacant job's function be performed by a volunteer or a staff member outside of the department?

Every hospital manager's goal should be to hire, develop, and maintain the most cohesive, productive, and flexible staff possible. Careful staffing is extremely important in a smaller hospital, where service delivery volumes can vary greatly on a daily basis. Creativity and extreme open-mindedness are essential for a department manager's team if the department is to respond to the rapidly changing health care delivery system.

With the desired staff in place, a department manager can begin to improve productivity by studying the components of work. The manager should start by performing the following job analysis:

- Determine daily work requirements.
- Identify the skill level necessary for each function.
- Determine which tasks should be performed immediately, and prioritize tasks that can wait.
- Make sure departmental staff have the tools needed to perform their jobs. Supplies and equipment must be readily available, and equipment must be fully operational.
- Respond when departmental conditions or responsibilities change or when projects do not produce expected outcomes.

Flexible Staffing

As mentioned earlier, hospital staffing requirements can change on a daily basis. In a smaller hospital, staffing requirements can change hourly in some departments. Department managers must be prepared to flex staffing to maintain productivity during these fluctuations.

The ability to adjust staffing requires a thorough understanding of departmental operations. Flexing staffing to address changing volumes of activity requires a complete understanding of how staff time is actually spent. Equally important is evaluating who performs what work. After each department's needs are evaluated, the hospital as a whole can be evaluated. Gathering facts concerning staffing requirements can be accomplished by using a two-step process.

Step 1: Identifying Responsibilities and Functions

In identifying departmental responsibilities and functions, an outside consultant has an advantage. Department managers can perform evaluations, too, as long as they can remain open-minded about reevaluating the functions and responsibilities for which they have been held accountable. The general responsibility of the department should be identified. All departmental tasks should then be listed. For example, patient baths, medication administration, and special procedures are common tasks for the medical/surgical department. Equally important is identifying which staff members perform these functions and what skill levels are required to perform each task. Knowing required skill levels will help the department managers delegate tasks to the lowest possible level.

Step 2: Determining Time Requirements

After identifying departmental functions, the next step is to determine how long each function takes to perform and how often each function occurs. This step may require the department manager or an outside party to monitor the time it takes staff to perform each function. During this process, the monitor should record findings to identify trends and compare performance among various staff members or work teams. It will also be important to record any disruptions that occur during the execution of each departmental function, such as telephone calls and interruptions by physicians, patients, and other hospital personnel.

The number of departmental tasks and the amount of time required for each one should be recorded. For medical/surgical nursing, recorded data might include the number of patient baths given each day, medications administered each shift, trips to the pharmacy and central supply for unstocked items each shift, special procedures performed per week, and phone calls to the floor per shift. It is important at this time to also identify who is doing each task.

The time requirement study should extend to the non–patient care areas of the hospital as well. For the food and nutritional services department, the tasks to record might be the number of patient meals prepared, nourishments passed, and special catering jobs completed per day. For the environmental services department, recorded tasks could include the amount of time it takes to clean one patient room, distribute linen for one nursing station, and wash and wax one hallway.

Once managers understand what is being done by whom and how long each function takes, they can begin to look for more efficient ways to perform departmental tasks. Sharing evaluation data with staff members and other department heads can help this process along. The best ideas for improved productivity will come from staff, not management. It is important to remember that they will be the ones who have to implement departmental improvements.

Daily Staffing

A good schedule balances work volume and staffing to meet the needs of patients, physicians, employees, and the hospital. Creating an effective daily schedule requires managers to *project* the next day's work load and *estimate* the next day's staffing. Managers must also *establish* the day's priorities, as well as *evaluate* daily activity patterns. The final step in creating an effective schedule is to *determine* employee responsibility.

If a manager finds the department's work load is increasing, the following steps should be taken before calling in the registry or hiring additional full-time staff members:

1. Keep departmental work load equal among staff and among shifts.
2. Simplify, put on hold, or eliminate noncritical projects and tasks.
3. Request help from staff of underutilized departments.
4. Increase part-time employee hours.
5. Use an established pool of on-call employees.
6. Flex schedule hours to address overload during certain shifts.
7. Consider overtime.

On the other hand, if a manager finds that work load is decreasing, the following steps should be taken before layoffs are initiated:

1. Schedule work and special projects that were previously delayed.
2. Assign staff to assist in other departments.
3. Train and educate staff to improve performance and satisfaction.
4. Cross-train employees to improve capabilities and flexibility.
5. Evaluate usage patterns and reschedule work.
6. If work load stays low, do not replace departing staff unless missing skill sets are absolutely essential.
7. Eliminate all overtime and contract help.
8. Allow employees to take days off without pay.
9. Reduce staff hours.

Staff Shifts and Rotations

Moving staff members into different roles for productivity, training, and motivational purposes is an excellent practice. Advanced planning, accompanied by personal counseling, is the key to staff shifting and rotating. Unplanned decisions often cost managers more in repercussions than what they had hoped to gain by the action. In rotating personnel, the following rules should be applied:

- Discuss staffing changes with involved parties ahead of time.
- Avoid forcing new assignments on individuals who are not sure they can perform the new tasks.
- Provide additional training to individuals performing new tasks.
- Give individuals a fair chance to perform new duties, but monitor the individual's performance.
- Recognize those who successfully make the adjustments.

Justification of Staff Increases

It may seem odd for a book on cost containment to discuss justifying a larger staff. However, many hospitals overemphasize staff control and cause bigger problems that, in the end, cost the hospital more money. Business office problems, medical record problems, and utilization review problems often result from too few staff working in critical areas. If department heads complain about departmental work loads, the complaints will be disregarded if the manager is unable to credibly support desired staffing needs. To justify a larger staff, managers should:

- Ask themselves whether they have made departmental functions as efficient as possible
- Support their overload position with facts
- Objectively compare today's heavier work load with the work loads of past periods
- Ask whether they can share someone from another department before hiring another employee
- Determine whether a part-time person can meet the department's needs, especially if it is impossible to hire a full-time employee

It is important to remember that when a supervisor seeks to add staff, management will look at the request with some level of scrutiny. Only when such close study reveals a well-run department will the request be given serious consideration. A less-than-justified request for additional staff will not be approved, and the request may not get an audience as easily the next time.

Staffing as the Key to Cost Containment

Staffing is the most important resource to control in any effort to contain costs. Staffing is the highest controllable cost item in the hospital budget, as well as the hospital's most valuable and scarce resource. Good employees are hard to come by, and their efforts should be directed toward areas where they can do the most good for the hospital. The examples provided in this chapter illustrate how other hospitals have been successful. Following the steps described in this chapter will help any hospital determine solutions to labor problems.

However, not every staffing issue can be answered by staff redesign. An efficient materials management function, incorporating purchasing and distribution systems, can also reduce the amount of unproductive staff time. Materials management and other cost-containment opportunities are discussed in the next chapter.

Note and Reference

1. An adjusted patient day is a calculation that factors outpatient business into the amount of hospital resources consumed relative to inpatient business. By dividing the hospital's inpatient revenue by total revenue, a factor for an adjusted patient day is determined. This factor is then multiplied by total patient days for that period's evaluated days. For example, if a hospital's total gross revenue for a month is $1 million and if the inpatient revenue is $500,000, with 300 total patient days for the month, then the total adjusted patient days for the month would be 600 ($1 million $\div$ $500,000 $\times$ 300 = 600).

2. Pounds, L. F., and Bauer, J. C. The future of the rural hospital: assessing the alternatives. *Trustee* 40(3):18–23, Mar. 1987.

Chapter 5

Managing Material Costs

Hospital supplies represent the second-highest hospital operating cost, after labor cost. Supply costs typically represent from 10 to 20 percent of gross patient service revenue. As a result, most hospitals have focused on this area in their cost-containment efforts. Usually, some success in controlling supply costs can be achieved without tremendous resistance from the medical staff or trauma within the hospital's organization.

Purchasing capital equipment demands a careful process as well. Selecting the most appropriate vendor, and skillfully negotiating specific inclusions during the acquisition process, can save a hospital significant amounts of money. Additionally, a hospital's materials management department can help control labor costs by efficiently using hospital personnel time when ordering and distributing materials.

Cost-containment efforts in materials management require the same basic strategy as other areas of cost containment. The hospital's administration and board must emphasize the importance of these cost-saving opportunities. Results will come only from the hospital staff's teamwork. Although the materials manager is central to this process, only through the voluntary actions of every hospital department can material costs be controlled. With so many opportunities to save money, managers and administrators might wonder where they should begin. The best place is where the least effort will bring the greatest level of results. A tool called ABC analysis helps the hospital set some priorities.

ABC Analysis

In the materials management process, the hospital should avoid majoring on the minors. With several thousand different supply items being purchased by the hospital, it is impossible to focus significant attention on each item and achieve effective results. An Italian economist, Alfredo

Pareto, developed a technique that can help the hospital establish priorities for the use of material management time—ABC analysis.

ABC analysis assumes that 10 percent of the inventory line items (the A items) represent 70 percent of total annual supply costs. Another 20 percent of the line items (the B items) represent 20 percent of the supply costs, and the remaining 70 percent of the inventory line items (the C items) represent only 10 percent of the hospital's annual supply costs. An ABC analysis attempts to isolate those few A and B items to which management should devote its cost-control attention. To perform an ABC analysis, four steps must be followed:

1. Identify the annual usage of each inventory item.
2. Determine the annual usage of each item in dollars by multiplying the number of times each item was purchased during the year by the unit price of the item.
3. List all items by ranking them in descending order from the highest annual dollar usage per item.
4. Identify which items listed represent the top 10 percent (the A items), the next 20 percent (the B items), and the remaining 70 percent (the C items) of hospital dollar usage.

Value Analysis

Once a hospital knows which inventory line items represent the majority of total annual supply costs, it must question whether resources are being spent wisely to acquire those items. Quality is conformance to requirements. In the case of equipment and supply purchases, the hospital determines its requirements and selects the materials that appear to be most capable of meeting those requirements. In other words, the hospital buys value.

Value analysis is one of the most objective techniques available in determining quality. It is an investigative process that first challenges the need for a product or service, then explores alternative ways to perform the same function, and finally studies the costs associated with the benefits received. Value analysis is a problem-solving approach that helps hospitals acquire the right goods and services for the right price consistent with the function that needs to be performed.

The following questions must be answered as part of a value analysis:

- What function(s) is required and how will the item or service perform this function?
- Is the item's cost appropriate to its usefulness?
- Are all of the item's features necessary to perform its stated functions? What bells and whistles are really not necessary?

- Based on competitive bids, is there any other vendor who offers the product or service at a lower price? If so, what are the differences in quality and reputation among the vendors?
- Has the hospital identified the most efficient and effective brand of a specific product to serve the required function?
- Can the service or product in question be accomplished in-house by using already-existing but underutilized hospital resources?

Volume Discounts

Once a hospital has clearly determined that an item or service is needed, the hospital's greatest opportunity to pay the lowest price rests with the power to negotiate volume discounts. Negotiating volume discounts can be a challenge for smaller hospitals that do not order supplies in enough volume to attract significant vendor discounts.

As a result, most smaller hospitals belong to an organization that negotiates contracts for a group of hospitals. Group purchasing organizations are usually established regionally and often consist of several hundred hospitals. Many of these organizations are established by the state hospital associations. Hospitals of the larger proprietary hospital corporations or health care systems (Hospital Corporation of America, HealthTrust, Volunteer Hospital Association, and so forth) usually have corporatewide negotiated purchasing contracts for member hospitals to use. Using such an organization's collective purchasing power, a hospital can often acquire supplies at significant cost savings. The group purchasing approach is a very effective way to contain costs, but there are limitations.

Although one vendor may hold a group's exclusive contract, there is often little or no assurance that member hospitals will use the vendor. For various reasons, hospitals continue to purchase selected items outside the group contracts. The exception to this trend is when proprietary chains institute compliance requirements for member hospitals. The lower the level of compliance, the less aggressive vendors will be in discounting product price.

Often a lack of compliance cannot be totally controlled by the hospital. Hospitals may have physicians who prefer particular items and may specify particular brand names when making orders. Hospital standardization efforts that include physician involvement will often reduce these problems and result in cost savings.

Product Standardization

Product standardization is as important in controlling supply costs as utilization management is in controlling resource consumption. A standardization program should analyze products to determine their effectiveness in meeting the operational requirements consistent with the hospital's mission to deliver patient care. Most hospitals have undertaken standardization programs, but it is not clear whether they have been effective.

The benefits of standardization are achieved through a well-planned and executed program. This program begins with the CEO's careful selection of standardization committee members. The standardization committee must establish and abide by its standards of success. Committee standards usually include three goals.

Quantities of inventory must be minimized by reducing the variety of products serving common functions. Often a hospital will stock several items that perform the same function because various physicians prefer different product brands. These duplications result in excess inventory carried because multiple minimum stock requirements compound the amount of redundant inventory, additional handling requirements, and higher unit prices resulting from fewer opportunities for economies of scale. Duplicate supply items should be identified and a full explanation developed for why the items are stocked. At a minimum, physicians who wish to use a particular brand should be able to justify to management or the standards committee the functional requirements for the added expense. An important aspect of this function is to "sell" the benefits of compliance with the hospital's group purchasing contracts to anyone who orders supplies and equipment.

New and improved products introduced for hospital purchase must be evaluated. Consistent with the concept of buying value, the standardization committee must determine possible measurable improvements in the quality of care, customer satisfaction, and cost efficiency through the testimony of other product users. It also becomes important for the committee to evaluate these issues in relation to their hospital's environment and patient volumes.

And third, the expense of educating and training personnel for new products must be reduced. When selecting a new product, the standards committee should negotiate to the greatest extent possible for the inclusion of user training and education into the item's purchase price. This negotiation is usually important to vendors as well because effective use of their products is what drives the continued ordering of the items.

Forming the Standardization Committee

Standardization only occurs through the efforts of several key hospital staff members. Although the CEO typically delegates responsibility for the supply and equipment buying process to the materials manager, many others are also involved. Every department in the hospital uses equipment and supplies and therefore should either routinely or occasionally attend standardization committee meetings. Furthermore, because physician ordering practices drive purchases, physician involvement and awareness are essential to the success of standardization efforts. As a result, the standardization committee should include medical staff members, as well as representatives of clinical and nonclinical hospital departments. If the CEO does not chair the standardization committee, the materials manager should.

Often the greatest challenge to product standardization is physician preference. For many hospital supplies and equipment, physicians are the ultimate consumers and have specific preferences. For example, some physicians may prefer one brand of analgesic over another. It is not surprising that vendor representatives spend time and money marketing to physicians. A member of the medical staff, therefore, should be appointed to the standardization committee by the medical staff president. This appointment should be considered part of the physician's fulfillment of hospital committee involvement.

It is in the physicians' best interest to participate in their hospital's standardization committee. The physicians' insight will help ensure that the committee's decisions meet the clinical needs of practicing physicians. Many physicians see committee involvement as an opportunity to receive valuable product orientation in an objective and discerning environment. Approached and executed correctly, standardization committee meetings may boast better physician attendance than many other hospital committee meetings. If physicians attending standardization committee meetings rotate each year, more will gain an appreciation of the cost and value considerations associated with supply and equipment selections and purchases.

Involving Hospital Employees

Through ABC analysis, a hospital will identify many patient care–oriented supplies (gauze, bed pads, sponges, and so forth), and the nursing department will certainly be affected by product standardization. Nurses can be helpful during the implementation of a standardization process, but they can also make the process more challenging. At times, the nursing floor receives free samples of new products from vendors. As the free stock is depleted, nurses sometimes order more quantities of the nonstocked items without going through the standardization procedure. By including nursing representatives on the standardization committee, these cost issues may be resolved. Committee representatives could include personnel from nurse management, the operating room staff, and the in-service education staff.

Other committee members to consider are representatives from the pharmacy, laboratory, and radiology departments, as well as any other areas significantly involved in the ordering of supplies. If a hospital wishes to economize on the number of hours spent attending meetings, a core group of committee members could be joined by representatives from specific departments when supplies from those departments are under discussion.

A natural management concern is that a continuous evaluation of products and services may lead to more items being purchased than might otherwise occur. Hospitals should not expect to see an acceptance rate any higher than 15 to 25 percent of items reviewed. And through this process, purchased items will have been carefully scrutinized, resulting in wiser buying decisions and lower costs.

Developing Policies and Procedures

The standardization committee must develop and follow specific policies and procedures. These policies and procedures should define who should be on the committee, how appointments to the committee should be made, when meetings should be held, and in what manner products should be reviewed. The following are some ideas to consider when developing standardization procedures:

- The committee should meet as often as standardization issues need to be covered. This may mean meeting as often as once a week when the committee begins its efforts and typically once a month after the standardization system is in place.
- The product review process must be well structured, beginning with a request for unstocked items needing evaluation that should be placed on the next meeting's agenda. Prior to the meeting, a form (similar to the example in figure 5-1) should be completed by the requesting individual or department. Items from all departments should be reviewed by the standardization committee with the exception of pharmacy items, which usually are reviewed by the pharmacy and therapeutics committee. It may not be practical for the committee to review perishable foods either.
- Upon hearing product presentations, the committee may accept the product, reject the product, or establish a product evaluation period, typically 30, 60, or 90 days.

Evaluating Products

Cost-effectiveness is the principal objective of the standardization process. Quantity requirements and quantity discounts should be considered when determining cost-effectiveness. The committee must explore possible opportunities to reduce unit costs, the number of purchase orders,

Figure 5-1.   Product Standardization Profile

Date: _____   Hospital Product Number: _____
Requested Product: _____
Manufacturer: _____
Supplied By: _____
Requested By: _____
Requested Item Will:
    ☐ Be an Additional Item
    ☐ Replace: _____
    ☐ Reduce Use of Another Item: _____
    ☐ Other: _____
Product Comparison:

Characteristics	Present Item	Requested Item
Supplier		
Usage per year		
Availability		
Charge to patient		
Packaging data		
Stock item		
Minimum order quantity		
Advantages		
Disadvantages		
Quantity on hand		
Cost per unit		
Net savings (or loss)		
Other		

Standardization Committee Action:
    ☐ Accepted
    ☐ Not Approved
    ☐ Approved for 30-Day Evaluation
    ☐ Approved for 60-Day Evaluation
    ☐ Approved for 90-Day Evaluation
    ☐ Tabled Pending Further Information
    ☐ Other: _____
Comments: _____
_____
_____
_____
Date: _____
Signature of Chairperson: _____

Source: Adapted from C. E. Housley. *Hospital Materiel Management.* Rockville, MD: Aspen Systems Corp., 1978, pp. 124–25.

and handling charges. Contract flexibility and the length of contract terms should also be discussed in cost-effectiveness studies.

Determining the quality of a product is also an important committee objective. Some specific criteria for determining quality include safety, storability, reusability versus disposability, and dependability. Examples of specific quality questions to ask include the following:

- Is the product free of mechanical and systemic hazards to the patient?
- If sterility is an issue, does the product permit sterile transfer from its package to the point where it is used?
- What is the product's shelf life? In a smaller hospital, utilization of a minimum order quantity for some items may be slow. For these items, the expense of spoilage could be significant if the shelf life is not consistent with the anticipated rate of demand. If the product's shelf life is significantly shorter than the use rate for the minimum order, other alternatives should be considered.
- Can the product be easily stored? If not, what are the special storage considerations and the associated cost? Smaller hospitals do not usually have large amounts of storage space. As new items are considered for purchase, the potential of a stockless inventory for the item will make the product more attractive. On the other hand, the cost required to add storage capacity to maintain a product's inventory can detract from its value.
- Are there any environmental issues to be considered for a disposable product? Occupational Safety and Health Administration (OSHA) requirements have quickly gained significant importance in hospitals over the past several years. The vendor should provide the standardization committee with all environmental safety requirements.
- Most important, will the product do what the vendor claims? This question can be answered by checking with existing customers. An evaluation of product performance and service-related aspects of the product must be conducted.

Evaluating Service

The service-related aspects of the product are of utmost importance and must be included in the product evaluation. Questions must be answered to ensure that products will arrive on time and in the quantities expected and to guarantee that hospital employees will be able to use the product properly. The following are examples of service-related questions:

- Is the product readily available or on back order?
- How much time usually expires between the receipt of a purchase order and the delivery of the product?

- What is the extent of in-service education provided by the manufacturer, and is the training effective?
- What is the availability of maintenance and repair support for equipment purchases?

Answers should be obtained from other hospitals with enough hands-on experience to provide feedback about the realized benefits and usefulness of the product in question.

Communicating with Users

It is extremely important that representatives of the hospital staff are included in product evaluations. If users are not included in the decision-making process, they may not be as likely to use the product. The physicians and department members may also know alternative vendors with similar products that should be considered in the selection. Often, staff contributions can lead to a selection of better value.

An example of effective communications in the purchasing process occurred at a 47-bed hospital in Texas. The hospital needed to replace its radiographic/fluoroscopic unit, which was no longer dependable. The standardization committee asked one of its members to investigate replacement possibilities.

In discussing replacement possibilities with the staff radiologist, a specific brand name of equipment was immediately suggested. The investigating member was able to learn from the radiologist the qualities that set this brand of equipment apart from alternative products. The hospital's radiology technologist was then consulted. After compiling the technologist's needs, a comparison of the preferred equipment traits of the physician and the technologist was presented to both parties. In discussing the competing needs, the radiology department's revenue and usage from the previous year were also reviewed. Some interesting conclusions resulted.

The technologist identified an alternative brand that would perform all the necessary functions at a significantly lower price than the physician's preferred brand. During interviews with current users of both products, the durability and maintenance downtime was found to be less for the technologist's brand than for the physician's preferred brand. One emerging problem with the alternative brand was that the availability of service representatives within the hospital's region was not as good as the physician's preferred brand.

Even after the facts of the evaluation were presented to the radiologist, he still exhibited a preference for his recommended brand. The radiologist did, however, recognize that hospital funds for this expenditure were limited. The gridlock was broken when the radiology technologist discovered that the hospital could purchase a refurbished model of the physician's preferred brand at a fraction of a new model's cost.

The hospital purchased the refurbished equipment. The decision received the full endorsement of the staff radiologist and, therefore, the rest of the physicians on staff. Had the hospital arrived at the same purchasing conclusion without the radiologist's involvement, he might have felt the hospital was making an irresponsible buying decision in selecting the refurbished model. Instead, the radiologist applauded the committee's resourcefulness. Additionally, the radiology technologist was very proud of her input in the decision, and the hospital was able to save a substantial amount (more than $100,000) of its capital budget.

Establishing a Formulary

As well as supply and equipment purchases, hospitals have significant cost-control opportunities when making drug purchases. The standard drugs to be dispensed in the hospital are recommended by the pharmacy and therapeutics committee. However, typically it is the hospital pharmacist's responsibility to select suppliers and brand names. By establishing a formulary system, a hospital can support the pharmacist in cost containment.

A *formulary* is a list of drugs that includes specifications of how those drugs should be used. These specifications may be no more than daily dosage rates, but may extend to cautions, warnings, restrictions, or pharmacology. A formulary system is organized by a committee composed primarily of practitioners that evaluates the therapeutic credentials of competing drug products. The system also requires the committee to periodically publish authorized preparations, procedures for drug list revision, and methods of communicating these revisions to physicians, nurses, pharmacists, and administrative staff. Additionally, a formulary may include guidelines for the use of nonformulary drugs.

A formulary is a helpful tool in containing unit drug costs, but managers and medical staff must still closely monitor the amounts of drug prescriptions purchased, as well as the prescriptions' appropriateness. A pharmacist's ability to influence the medical staff's prescribing habits remains a critical component in pharmacy cost containment.[1]

Inventory Management

There are two kinds of inventory: official and unofficial. *Official inventory* is brought into a hospital or storeroom, counted, and controlled until it is dispensed to a using department. It is assigned an inventory account number and is charged to the using department when dispensed. Once official inventory supplies have been expensed and dispensed to be stored or used in the user departments, they become *unofficial inventory.*

Typically, minimum and maximum amounts are used when reordering. Official inventory is physically counted at least once per year and entered into the hospital's financial statement as an asset. Through accounting for purchases less issues, the hospital accounting department attempts to reasonably balance this official figure during the fiscal year.

Monitoring the Turnover Rate

For inventory management purposes, it is important to know how quickly inventory turns over in a hospital. The number of times total inventory dollars are issued and replaced is the *inventory turnover rate*. This rate is calculated by dividing supply expense by the ending inventory for a period. For example, if a hospital's inventory at the end of a fiscal year is $70,000 and supply expenses for the year are $630,000, the inventory turnover rate would be: $630,000 ÷ $70,000 = 9 times.

Developing Order Points and Par Levels

Beyond monitoring the inventory turnover rate, hospital management often focuses its attention on supply and equipment prices. Total cost containment requires having the right quantities at the right price in the right place at the right time. Achieving total cost containment begins with the development of proper order points and par levels for each supply item.

Order Points

The use of order points helps hospitals determine when to order additional supply units. A hospital's materials manager uses several factors to calculate an inventory level that will satisfy expected demand for an item from the time an order is placed to when it arrives (the lead time). When an issue of stock causes inventory on hand and on order to drop below this predetermined level, the hospital reorders that item (unless the hospital no longer wishes to stock the item).

The *order point* is the level of stock required in inventory to support a hospital during the replenishing time without outages under historic conditions. It is the expected lead time for reordering expressed as the rate of demand for that item. The order point, then, must incorporate the time necessary to receive an ordered item, as well as the number of item issues anticipated during that time. The average lead time should be calculated using figures from no less than the preceding five order periods. For example, if the lead time in days for the preceding five order periods is 6, 8, 4, 5, and 7, the average lead time would be 6 days.

Consideration must be given to the longest lead time involved. Order point calculation assigns an added weight to the longest period, subtracting the average lead time from the longest lead time, and adding half of this difference to the average to reflect a more accurate lead time. This calculation can be illustrated with the preceding example. The longest lead time, 8 days, subtracted from the average lead time, 6 days, leaves a difference of 2 days. If half the difference, or 1 day, is added to the average, the final average lead time for the item would be 7 days.

Another factor to consider is the time between requisition generation and actual order placement. In many cases, the requisition and purchase order will be cut on the same day. However, there may be delays in the ordering process due to minimum dollar requirements, batching of purchase orders to reduce ordering time and freight costs, and so forth, and these delays should be considered in the ordering process. Therefore, lead time calculations should be based on the period from the date an item is requisitioned to the date an item is received.

Estimating demand for an item during the needed lead time requires a second calculation. One method of calculating this demand is to divide the total annual issues by 365 days and multiply this average by the calculated lead time. This approach, however, does not consider trending, seasonal, or daily changes in issuing patterns for the item. A more accurate approach uses an item's issue history corresponding to the dates currently being used for lead time calculations. If previous year issues corresponding to the lead time days calculated in the preceding example were 5, 9, 3, 7, and 11, the average lead time demand would be 7 issues. If the high issue amount is treated in a similar fashion to the longest lead time calculation, the order point quantity is calculated as follows:

Highest issue amount   11
Average issue amount   7
Difference   4
Half of difference   2

Order point quantity = 7 + 2 = 9

When the stocked inventory in the hospital drops below 9 items, the hospital places its order.

Par Levels

A *par-level program* is used to accomplish two objectives: it brings user department inventories under the control of the hospital materials manager, and it takes the function of requisitioning supplies and managing inventory levels away from user departments. In par-level programs, the materials manager works with user departments in establishing standard maximum item quantities for the various units. These items are typically stocked in the user departments, utilizing existing shelving and cabinets. Supplies are checked periodically by the storeroom personnel and refilled to maximum stock levels established for each item. The frequency of stock replenishment is adjusted to meet each department's needs. For example, restocking for a nursing department may be required daily, but a radiology department may need to be replenished only once per week.

When first establishing a par-level system, the hospital materials management department must quickly gain the confidence of each user department. User departments will be concerned that stock levels may not be sufficient to handle demand between requisitions. Initially, it is wise to establish liberal stock maximums to reduce the possibility for any stockouts. Once a history of stock levels has been established, par levels can be reduced as appropriate.

Using a Supply Cart Exchange System

A major limitation to the par-level system will be the availability of adequate storage shelves and cabinets. Additionally, stocking department shelves is time-consuming for materials management personnel.

An alternative to the par system is to use supply carts in an exchange system. All the supplies for a department are placed on a cart (or carts). Supply levels are established according to par-level-system guidelines. At least two carts are required per user department. One cart can then be stocked from the storeroom while a department is pulling supplies from the other. The full cart is taken to the floor every day to replace the depleted cart. The depleted cart is then filled to the established maximum levels and sent back to the floor as the next day's full cart.

There are several advantages to the exchange cart approach. Materials management personnel are more productive, spending most of their time in the hospital storeroom instead of stocking supplies on the floors. Accountability for supplies is also improved because carts are consistently checked prior to the next day's exchange.

Examples of departments where exchange carts can be used include medical/surgical nursing, surgery, emergency, and physical therapy. Potentially prohibitive factors include the actual expense associated with purchasing the carts and whether the physical plant layout will restrict cart movement between the storeroom and user departments.

Establishing a Stockless Inventory

The smaller hospital should also consider establishing a stockless inventory for all appropriate items. The object of a stockless inventory is to reduce redundant inventory in the departments and in the storeroom.

This approach is focused on those items primarily used by only one or two departments. Laboratory and radiology are examples of specialized departments well suited for the stockless inventory approach.

There are several advantages to the stockless inventory approach. Valuable storeroom space is reclaimed. Cash flow is improved because less money is required to maintain inventory. Responsibility for effective supply cost containment is placed on the manager of the user department. And finally, the hospital is able to put more emphasis on controlling unofficial inventory.

A stockless inventory approach is accomplished by delivering ordered supplies directly to user departments instead of to the storeroom. The four steps for implementing a stockless inventory are the following:

1. Identify storeroom items being maintained for only one or two departments.
2. Combine these items with other items not being stocked in the storeroom and perform an analysis of usage and supplier lead time.
3. Establish quotas for each item in conjunction with its user department. Management should allow flexible quotas so that adjustments can be made based on actual ordering results.
4. Create a routine order cycle and a special requisition form to help user departments order through the materials management department.

Periodic ordering for stockless inventory is done at fixed intervals instead of through the reorder point approach. Periodic ordering is a simpler and preferred ordering method for stockless inventory. Usually the amount of stockless inventory for each item is equal to the amount needed for a two-week period. This inventory level allows inventory for that item to turn over 26 times per year. In some cases, items may move too slowly to turn over every two weeks, and so flexibility is also important.

The use of a stockless inventory affects many areas within a hospital. It brings the hospital materials manager in direct contact with the entire management structure. Stockless inventory eliminates at least one level of the materials management function, leading to fewer problems and greater productivity in the supply function. It also requires less paperwork and provides better control over unofficial inventory. Most important, stockless inventory can have a significant effect by reducing overall inventory and promoting the use of vendors identified through the standardization process. A stockless inventory should be considered for as many hospital items as possible.

Capital Equipment Management

The materials management function for purchasing equipment differs significantly from purchasing supplies in several ways. A smaller hospital's capital budget is usually small and consequently only a few capital purchases are made each year. One oversight in the acquisition process can prove disastrous. Purchases from vendors with whom a hospital has little previous experience can add even more risk to making selections. Unlike most supplies, equipment purchases may also include the negotiation of warranty and service agreements. And almost certainly, the final equipment selection will require board approval.

Because of these differences, extra consideration must be given to the capital equipment purchasing process. Many of the steps discussed in this chapter relating to value analysis and standardization should be followed, but smaller hospitals should also consider the following procedures when developing their own equipment-purchasing policies:

1. Each department should submit equipment purchase requests to the hospital finance department (or budget committee) for consideration in the hospital's capital budget. When approved by the hospital CEO, the item's name, reason for purchase, and estimated purchase cost should be specified in the annual equipment budget.
2. After approval, the administration should meet with the affected department heads to determine the item's projected purchase date.
3. As the purchase date approaches, a requisition should be submitted by the user department to the materials management department, which then requests quotations from every acceptable source.
4. Discussions and meetings (as discussed earlier in this chapter in the standardization section) should occur among the standardization committee, representatives of the medical staff, and the department head(s) who will be using the equipment.
5. The vendors' quotations and a recommendation for purchase selection should be given to the CEO. Approval authority with a dollar limit (for example, $15,000) should also be given to the CEO. Any items over that limit would require approval of the hospital's board of trustees.
6. The materials manager should notify the submitting vendor that the dollar amount quoted will be the total financial commitment for the purchase. Any additional costs above that amount will be paid by the supplier.
7. Hospital policy should state that payment is made in full upon installation and acceptance of the equipment by the hospital. The

vendor may want partial payment prior to that time, but the materials manager should usually be able to avoid payment by stating the hospital's policy. When payment is made after installation and approval, delivery and installation are more likely to be timely. The hospital will also accrue more interest on its money as well!

8. Purchased equipment should be inspected upon receipt by a skilled technician (a biomedical engineer, for example) from the hospital. The inspector should look for damage or operational concerns and assess whether the equipment meets local and regulatory standards. All operating manuals should also be reviewed during this inspection.

9. All equipment purchases should be free on board (FOB) to the hospital. The hospital should avoid partial shipments to minimize the chance that components will be lost in transit.

Benefits of Effective Materials Management

Through effective materials management, a smaller hospital can reduce its supply, capital equipment, and payroll costs. Effective materials management requires the active involvement of not only the materials manager but also administrators, user departments, and medical staff. The hospital CEO can set the tone for materials management efforts by enforcing policy, maintaining accountability, and influencing the thinking of others. The most challenging and the most critical element of success in this area, however, is changing the habits of the medical staff, the subject of the next chapter.

Reference

1. Rowland, H. S., and Rowland, B. L. *Hospital Management: A Guide to Departments*. Rockville, MD: Aspen Systems Corp., 1984, pp 254–56.

Bibliography

Rucker, D. T. Effective formulary development: which direction? *Topics in Hospital Pharmacy Management* 1(1):29–45, May 1981.

Chapter 6

Working with the Medical Staff

The 1980s brought about significant changes in hospital–physician relationships. There has been unprecedented concern about health care expenditures and, most recently, a call for demonstrated quality in the delivery of that care. As much as hospital administrators may try to reduce departmental costs by making managers more responsible for financial performance, only a physician can admit and discharge patients and order services. Every major hospital expenditure is, therefore, controlled more by physicians than by anyone else in the hospital.

Trends in the 1990s will continue to focus health care cost control and outcome measurement on physicians. Employers and third-party payers are already collecting data to profile the performance of physicians (as well as hospitals) related to costs, severity of illness, and outcomes. Because the sickest and most resource-consumptive patients are treated in a hospital, the physician's performance in the hospital will clearly be the one most scrutinized by purchasers of health care services. Controlling costs and continuously improving quality in the hospital is the joint responsibility of physicians, members of the board of trustees, and managers. If hospitals and physicians do not seize this decade's opportunity to set standards for controlling costs and improving quality, payers will set those standards for them.

Physicians need to change their practice habits, and hospitals need to foster that change. Whether they are dealing with improving medical record documentation, altering treatment protocols, or wrestling with discharge planning issues, hospital administrators must look at ways to change existing habits. This change will only be accomplished over the long term by influencing physician thinking. If a hospital attempts to directly control physician performance on a case-by-case basis, the levels of expected value in health care delivery will not be achieved. Physicians, managers, and board members must together undertake careful strategic planning and demonstrate a willingness to devote needed resources for developing and managing a collaborative improvement program. Controlling costs and improving outcomes by changing behaviors and systems must be viewed not as penalizing individuals but rather as working together toward common goals.

Efforts to Change Physician Behavior

Various studies have shown that there are significant differences in the way physicians treat patients with the same diagnosis. Historically, hospitals have failed to develop standards of care based on diagnosis and treatment protocols. The increased attention to controlling health care costs and the desire to improve outcomes have inspired several efforts to create programs intended to change the way physicians use medical services. Some of these efforts are being initiated by hospitals and medical groups. Others are being developed by organizations representing employers. Still other efforts are being developed by third-party payers, health maintenance organizations, and various other managed care organizations. Successful programs involve physicians from the beginning and focus on confidential efforts to change behavior and systems to address control-of-cost and quality-of-care issues.

The factors associated with physicians' use of services are complex. Personal preferences, patient characteristics, coding and documentation of the correct principal and secondary diagnoses, and availability of ancillary service resources (especially a concern in smaller, rural facilities) are just some of the reasons why similar cases may be treated differently. Even when physicians within a community have similar practice patterns, there may still be opportunities to improve the way the entire group is providing care. In the area of efficiency and cost-effectiveness, all that many physicians who have homogeneous patterns can say for sure is that they are "just as expensive in delivering care as the next guy." From a payer's perspective, that claim may not be good enough.

Most physicians are not very fond of hospital representatives, whether it be the CEO, the utilization review coordinator, or anyone else, who approach them with questions about their overutilization of services. Most physicians are very concerned about losing their autonomy in practicing medicine. When approached by management, the physician's answer most often given to overutilization questions is "my patients are sicker," a phrase that means in doctorese "go away."

However, there may be a better, less-threatening way to approach physicians about utilization. If management could persuade physicians to collect, analyze, and present performance information to their peers—and if this information could be presented in a less-aggressive manner, perhaps comparing physician profiles for patients with similar conditions—physicians might be more likely to listen. When this presentation is combined with information valuable to the physician's practice, the chance for a collaborative effort to improve rises dramatically.

Physician Profiles

The objective in improving overutilization is to help physicians understand that their utilization habits are significantly different from either the habits of other staff physicians or established standards of treatment for specific diagnoses, or both. There are several steps the hospital should take toward achieving this objective.

Comparing Apples to Apples

The first step is to compare data pertaining to charges (and variable costs, if available) as well as length of stay per diagnosis-related group (DRG) for each physician on staff. To obtain meaningful data a hospital must compare apples to apples. This can be accomplished by distinguishing patient severity for a sample of cases reviewed within a DRG or segregating cases within the study. The way the hospital decides to collect such data depends on how much the hospital is willing to spend on information.

Through the use of software or outside services, the hospital can develop refined DRG information that groups severity of cases within a specific DRG. Physician profiles can then be compared based on a severity-adjusted factor within the DRG. For example, based on the number and complexity of diagnoses within a specific DRG, each of three physicians' profiles is awarded a severity-adjusted coefficient for the dollar value of reported charges. The physician with the highest severity of cases within the DRG is given a coefficient of 0.87, and the physician with the lowest severity is given a coefficient of 1.21. The third physician treats patients considered to be of average severity for the DRG and is therefore awarded a 1.00 coefficient. These severity coefficients are then multiplied by actual charges or costs to determine severity-adjusted profiles. This comparison process involves not only investment for sorting and analysis services, but also additional coding requirements for the hospital's medical record personnel.

With the existing challenge to place and keep skilled medical record coders, the smaller hospital may want to explore less-costly methods of comparing data. One of these alternatives is to segregate the cases of similar patients within a DRG. In this process, certain cases would be identified for exclusion from the profiled sample because of their infrequent occurrence. Although cases are excluded for many different reasons, usually the profiled sample will exclude cases of very low severity and very high severity within a given DRG. Patient classification criteria might include patient age, discharge status, the number of body systems affected, and the number of patient comorbidities and complications.

An example of how these criteria would be used to exclude a case among Medicare patients treated within DRG 89 (simple pneumonia and pleurisy with comorbidity or complication) would look like this:

65-year-old female
Discharged to home without need for home health care
Diagnoses: right upper lobe pneumonia; urinary tract infection

This case would be considered of low severity because the patient is relatively young among the Medicare population and would not need skilled nursing as a condition of being discharged and because there are only two body systems (respiratory and urinary) involved and one comorbid condition (the urinary tract infection).

The following is an example of a high-severity case that would be excluded from a sample profile of patients treated within DRG 89:

92-year-old male
Discharged to skilled nursing facility
Diagnoses: right upper lobe pneumonia; congestive heart failure; chronic obstructive pulmonary disease; hyponatremia; malnutrition; decubitus ulcer, right heel

In this case, the patient is very old and he will need skilled nursing care after discharge. In addition, his diagnoses cover five body systems (respiratory, circulatory, renal, metabolic, and skin) as well as representing five comorbid conditions. The complications and comorbidities (CCs) listed are those recognized by Medicare for potential payment change under the DRG payment system, and treating those CCs identified will necessitate an increase in length of stay by at least one day in 75 percent of the cases.

The cases falling between these two extremes would be included in the sample profile. The cost information for these cases should be trended over a period of time to minimize the chance of one or two cases misrepresenting a physician's general treatment practices. This information can be presented to physicians in a format similar to the one illustrated in figure 6-1.

Preparing and Analyzing Profiles

When physician profiles are being prepared, it is important that enough detail be included so that physicians can understand exactly what should

Figure 6-1. Sample Departmental Physician Cost Profiles

| | | | | Average Ancillary Departmental Charges | | | |
| | Number | Total Average | | | | | Length |
Physician	of Cases	Charge	ICU	Lab	Pharmacy	Radiology	of Stay
A	17	$4,385	—	$1,258	$1,539	$152	3
B	11	2,309	$ 50	294	342	98	5
C	5	4,808	125	1,608	330	508	8
D	5	1,879	—	165	216	207	3
E	10	4,111	750	1,123	618	64	7

DRG X
Fiscal Year 1991

be changed in order to improve their profiles. Ideally, this profile information should detail specific tests being performed by physicians. Unfortunately, this level of information is not always readily available in smaller hospitals. When detailed information is not available, management should begin with gathering department-level information.

The departmental cost information illustrated in figure 6-1 is based on reported charges. As mentioned in chapter 3, controlling costs in a smaller hospital has been a strategic issue for a long time, and an effective budget and budgeting process are typically the best tools available in controlling costs. Because the issue of how better to use the available time of skilled personnel is more important to smaller hospitals than the actual cost of one procedure versus another, the hospital often does not have the elaborate procedural cost information that a larger hospital might have.

Reported charges will be the best available information in a smaller hospital when elaborate cost information is not available. With the revenue importance that charge capture has had to hospitals, this information is usually readily available. When a hospital has completely and accurately captured its charges, it can explore possible resource management opportunities. If a hospital does not know how well it is capturing its charges, hospital management should consider the use of an outside consultant to assist in this process. Special studies can be initiated with the assistance of consultants to gather measures of service intensity at the department, diagnosis, or DRG level.

The most readily available hospital cost-to-charge ratios are reported through the Medicare/Medicaid Cost Report. In Worksheet C, Part 1 and Part 2, hospitals are to report an accumulation of all direct and indirect costs for each department. These costs are then compared to gross charges for inpatient and outpatient services. These reported data are used to determine specific portions of cost-based reimbursement. Although Medicare reimbursement methodology continues to shift away from payment based on cost, the reporting of cost data continues to be a requirement. These data, however, do not include all costs that are considered nonallowable for reimbursement by Medicare and Medicaid. In using these data for cost profiles, consultation should occur with the hospital's reimbursement experts to fully understand the extent and nature of these data.

By reviewing costs on a departmental basis, the hospital and its physicians can begin to develop a clinical pathway for the DRG previously reviewed. In so doing, however, clinical pathways must be connected to the achievement of optimum clinical outcomes, not merely to the costs of treatment. Cost reductions and improvements in clinical outcomes are generally complementary, not contradictory. Significant cost reductions can be achieved in part by reducing length of stay, but reductions in unnecessary variations in care patterns have more influence.

By reviewing the departmental costs shown in figure 6-1, it becomes clear that physician C's total charges are significantly higher than the other physicians' charges, possibly because the other physicians handle fewer cases with this DRG. On the other hand, physician B seems to be using either fewer or less-costly lab tests than physician A or physician E. Physician D appears to be the most cost-effective physician in treating these cases. After comparing these physicians' cost profiles, the data reviewed provide physicians and management with a direction to investigate even further the services being ordered and why they are necessary.

Management should expect a challenge to the accuracy of the physician profile data. Before presenting the profiles, management and at least one physician should carefully review the accuracy of variances and the method of determining variances. Questions to be asked during this review should include: Are we accurately capturing all charges associated with the case? Is the cost-to-charge ratio correct for cost information, or is it biased for optimum reimbursement?

The hospital should resist the temptation to focus attention on the physician with the highest utilization rates. This attention will most likely result in defensiveness and offers little promise for improvement. The hospital's objective should be to bring all the physicians closer to the exemplary performer, with an understanding that each physician will not accept the idea of conformance at the same rate.

Physician conformance will increase over time. Some physicians will lead the process, others will follow; that is, as more physicians see the importance of cost containment, they will induce others to conform as well. Although the hospital CEO should place significant emphasis on the importance of utilization information for both the hospital and its physicians, peer pressure among physicians is much more powerful than anything hospital management could ever hope to achieve directly. Formal physician leaders (the chief of the medical staff, the vice-president of medical affairs, the department chairpersons, and so forth) should work with management in achieving "buy-in" with a few of the informal physician leaders (that is, influential physicians on staff such as respected clinicians and physician advocates). Eventually, more physicians will recognize that monitored cost performance is a fact of managed medical life. Hospital and physician costs will eventually be more effectively controlled as a result of these efforts.

Sharing Cost and Charge Data with Physicians

Should cost data be shared with the medical staff? If they are, how should the physicians be approached? Many hospital CEOs have been very concerned about physicians' reactions to the presentation of cost data. This concern stems from hospital management's view of physicians as "customers" who control the flow of patients to the hospital. However, more and more physicians are also becoming interested in knowing cost information. With reduced payments and greater emphasis on utilization review from Medicare and other third-party payers, physicians are more closely examining the efficiency and appropriateness of treatment within their practices.

In the evolving managed care environment, control of patient traffic is moving away from the physician and toward the employer and managed care entity. Like physicians, employers and managed care organizations are increasingly viewed as customers who expect improvements in costs and outcomes and who must be satisfied if hospitals are to meet their objectives. Physicians must join the hospital in satisfying these new customers.

The sensitivity of physicians to cost information is, however, something to respect. Regardless of whether physicians control patient activity or not, cooperation is the only way to achieve improvements in cost-effectiveness. The hospital must carefully develop a communication plan with an initial objective of enabling the physicians and hospital to understand problems and improvement opportunities in the same way.

Keeping the Communication Simple

When the hospital begins sharing cost and charge information with physicians, education on hospital reimbursement and accounting basics should be included. Typically, physicians have not understood the difference between hospital charges and hospital payments. Also, many physicians do not understand the difference between fixed and variable or direct and indirect costs.

Regardless of the detailed cost or charge information available to present to physicians in their profiles, the one thing physicians will easily understand is unit utilization. For example, if one physician always uses a complete blood count (CBC) with white blood cell differential count, while other physicians are able to manage equally sick patients with fewer, less-costly tests, it is more likely that this testing information, rather than cost figures, will influence higher-utilizing physicians toward a change in practice patterns.

Approaching Physicians

All hospital employees and volunteers who are responsible for working with physician profiles must be trained in effective ways to approach physicians with this information. Ideally, physician volunteers should be involved. In addition, hospital employees with a clinical background could be enlisted to discuss reasonable utilization alternatives with the medical staff.

The hospital may initially develop profiles only for those physicians who are interested. Interested physicians usually have other incentives beyond helping the hospital reduce costs. For example, profiles will assist those physicians in identifying opportunities to be more efficient in providing care. The profiles will also help them ensure they are treating patients in an acceptable manner consistent with the patients' diagnoses. Once a few physicians demonstrate the value of profile information, other physicians may become more interested in the profiling process. Some hospitals have even used a physician to approach the other physicians, which can at times be effective and well accepted.

Ensuring Management Support

Staff members and volunteers working with physicians must have management's support. Even though the physicians may have expressed an interest in receiving profile data, they are not accustomed to nurses or other hospital representatives presenting information that might suggest suboptimal practice patterns. Physicians accept such information more readily from their peers, including department chairpersons. Nevertheless, physicians, like most people, do not like to receive negative information or information that presents them as different from their colleagues.

Because physicians may at any time choose to send their patients to another hospital, administration will be tempted to ease off physicians who have variant profiles and are easily offended. Administration should be aware that these problems may occur, and the potential consequences should be weighed before anyone approaches a physician.

If a hospital is going to back off when a physician complains about the presentation of profiles, then administrators should not waste time and money on developing the profiles in the first place. Nor should the hospital frustrate and waste the talents of those responsible for creating and presenting the profiles.

Supplying Correct Data

A hospital must be certain that comparative profile data are accurate. Problems begin with inaccurate ICD-9-CM coding and inappropriate documentation in patient medical records to support the coding. The ICD-9-CM codes describe diagnoses associated with a patient's case; they are intended to describe why a patient received specific treatment. Medicare and a growing number of other payers have adopted a method of determining a flat payment for hospitals based on ICD-9-CM codes grouped into DRGs.

Under DRG grouping and payment methodology, a hospital may be paid more when more diagnoses are reported. Typically, these payment increases are based on assigning a change in principal diagnosis or adding a secondary diagnosis that supports payment for more severe cases. Once a DRG is optimized for payment, no matter how many more diagnoses are listed, the DRG and related payment remain the same.

Many hospitals still are not accurately documenting and coding. In other cases, a hospital may accurately code for optimal payment, but does not complete medical record documentation. Medical record personnel can only code what has been documented in the record.

The best way to obtain the most accurate diagnoses is to document the patient's medical record during the patient's length of stay. This concurrent approach requires a clinical understanding of the case as well as an understanding of how to code DRGs. A sample pneumonia case can be used to demonstrate what the concurrent approach can do to improve the accuracy of DRG selection.

A 68-year-old male arrived in the hospital emergency room with complaints of a fever, shortness of breath, and a productive cough. Vital signs indicated a temperature of 102 degrees, a pulse rate of 102 beats per minute and regular, and 24 respirations per minute. Arterial blood gases were within normal limits, but a chest X ray revealed a left lower lobe pneumonia. Various tests were ordered to identify further refinement of the diagnosis, including a sputum culture, blood culture, urine culture, complete blood count with white blood cell differential count, a chemistry profile 23, and a urinalysis. At that time, the diagnosis stated that the patient was admitted with a working diagnosis of left lower lobe pneumonia, DRG 90, and simple pneumonia without CC—Medicare relative case weight of 0.7282.[1]

On day 2 of the patient's hospitalization, the utilization manager observed that the patient's urinalysis indicated an abnormal level of white blood cells and bacteria present. The nurses had documented that the patient was complaining of painful urination. The utilization manager placed a note to the physician in the medical record highlighting the abnormal lab results and asking whether the physician felt the patient had a urinary tract infection.

On day 3, the physician addressed the urinalysis in his progress notes, indicating that he believed the patient already had the urinary tract infection (UTI) at the time of admission. The working DRG was changed to left lobe pneumonia with the comorbid condition (a secondary diagnosis) of UTI. This diagnosis qualified for DRG 89, simple pneumonia with CC and a Medicare relative case weight of 1.1658.

On day 4, the utilization manager found that the blood culture was negative. However, the sputum culture was positive for *Klebsiella* pneumonia. Again, a note was placed in the medical record asking the physician to address the diagnosis if he agreed with the laboratory findings.

On day 5, the utilization manager found that the physician had agreed with the lab report findings and had changed the diagnosis to *Klebsiella* pneumonia. The patient was discharged and sent home. The final DRG assigned for the case was DRG 79, Respiratory Infections and Inflammations, with CC. The Medicare relative case weight was 1.7813.

Depending on how cost profiles are being established, the accuracy of assigning the DRG affects the case's cost profile. The difference among cost profiles in the previous example are illustrated in figure 6-2. Assuming that the cost of treating the pneumonia patient would not have changed due to the need to treat the existing comorbid conditions, the case weight-adjusted cost profile for the example changes dramatically depending on which DRG is assigned.

As the hospital examines its physician practice patterns on a DRG-by-DRG basis, valuable information concerning cost variances will surface. This DRG-by-DRG study will often provide the hospital and physician with more information than would have been available through only monitoring overall length of stay. As this information is examined,

Figure 6-2. Sample Cost Profiles for Three DRGs

DRG	Case Weight	Total Case Cost	Case Weight-Adjusted Cost
90	0.7282	$5,000	$6,866
89	1.1658	$5,000	$4,289
79	1.7813	$5,000	$2,807

the physicians and the hospital can begin to explore opportunities for improvement.

The physician cost profiles in figure 6-1 display varying levels of cost and length of stay for the same DRG. For the cost profiles to be relevant for comparison, the data being compared must be limited to similar cases only. In figure 6-1, the only cases included are those with the same outcome (discharged home) and those performed by physicians who had treated at least five such cases during the calendar year. Those cases that required an extended stay beyond the Medicare maximum stay (outliers) are not included. To avoid embarrassing the physicians involved, each physician's profile is represented by a letter instead of a name. Each physician knows only the letter that corresponds to his or her individual profile. The physician shown as C has an average length of stay of 8 days and the highest cost per case. It is interesting to note, however, that physician A has a higher cost profile than physician E, even though physician A's average length of stay for this DRG is four days less than that of physician E.

These data serve several purposes. The data can be shared among the physicians so that they can understand how their profiles compare with those of other staff physicians. The hospital can also begin to study the physician with the lowest cost profile to determine whether this pattern of treatment would be a reasonable guideline (that is, a critical, or clinical, pathway) to be used by other physicians treating similar cases. This study should focus on clinical processes that yield good clinical and cost outcomes.

To aid in the development of clinical pathways, the Division of Quality Resources of the American Hospital Association can provide examples of clinical practice guidelines (also known as practice parameters) that can be modified and implemented in hospitals. Such modifications are crucial, because any successful strategy involving clinical processes must be tailored to the clinical, managerial, and political circumstances of each individual hospital and medical staff.

However, the hospital may not want to set up pathways for their physicians to follow at all. The sharing of individual cost profiles with physicians may be enough to influence their own interest in more effective methods of treatment. The data should bring to the medical staff's attention the fact that practice habits need to be reviewed and opportunities for improvement should be discussed.

It is important to remember that financial and clinical results from working with physician profiles will probably not be recognized immediately. Significant time must be allowed for data to be compiled and analyzed. Nor should the hospital expect to be successful in getting physicians to immediately follow altered treatment protocols. Physicians must be allowed enough time to observe trends and draw their own conclusions based on the data available to them.

Using Profiles in the Credentialing Process

Perhaps physician defensiveness about profiles stems from their fear that profile information will be used against them during the credentialing process. Financial data, such as figures used to determine the minimum and maximum numbers of specialists needed on staff, are already used at some hospitals. In addition, as exclusive provider arrangements are struck between employers and hospital–physician organizations, the employers may require some level of economic credentialing.

The question often arises whether economic credentialing is legal. The answer will depend, in part, on how this concept is defined by each facility and, in part, on the facility's legal status. For example, a non-profit, tax-exempt hospital might assert that its board of trustees has a fiduciary obligation to ensure that the hospital, a charitable asset, is not "wasted" by inefficient business and/or medical practices. Likewise, proprietary facilities might assert a similar duty on behalf of their share-holders. In either case, a central theme of economic credentialing is to relate credentialing decisions to the quality of medical performance of each practitioner.

Because this question includes so many variables, it is hard to recommend that a smaller hospital become the pioneer of economic credentialing at this time. This concept is likely to evolve, and hospitals should look instead toward attempts to influence thinking rather than to control results.

Physician Bonding Techniques

There are several methods for a hospital to develop a closer relationship with its physicians. The continuing changes to the payment system will require more teamwork among providers to meet the requirements of those who pay for health care. This will mean more joint ventures and other arrangements involving physicians and hospitals.

Several legal limitations on joint ventures exist. Fraud and abuse legislation, the corporate practice of medicine, and safe harbor regulations have all helped to better define the parameters under which joint ventures can be formed and operate. But these parameters should not prohibit formation of hospital–physician ventures. Ventures that focus on less-costly alternatives to care are likely to be welcomed.

Offering Financial Incentives

A change in financial incentives can be an effective way to promote efficient practice patterns. Research indicates that in health maintenance organizations with capitated plans, physicians show lower rates of in-patient and outpatient utilization. Physicians are less likely to refer a patient to another specialist within this environment.

Under the reform strategy of the American Hospital Association, health care providers are being encouraged to focus their attention on the establishment of community care networks. Such networks may help align physician, hospital, and patient incentives. It is recognized, however, that the alignment of these incentives can be very controversial and hence must be tailored to individual circumstances.

Sharing the Risk

Physicians tend to be averse to risk taking and look to the hospital to assume the risk of any venture or project. However, this attitude is changing. Medicare safe harbor requirements prescribe a specific amount of actual investment by physicians, and management requires some assurance of physician commitment to any joint ventures. In other arrangements, varying degrees of risk may be shared by physicians and others. But in all cases, risk must be proportional to reward and ventures must be selected on the basis of individual and community circumstances.

Offering Convenience

Convenience is probably the smaller hospital's greatest differential advantage with physicians. It is easier for both physicians and patients to get to a smaller local hospital. The drive is shorter, parking is easier, and it is simpler to find one's way around the facility. Because of its limited medical staff, a smaller hospital can usually be more effective in customizing scheduling for physicians, thus making it possible for physicians to see more patients in less time. Nurses in smaller hospitals are more likely to provide personal attention to patients and foster greater patient satisfaction with the entire hospital experience.

These are qualities smaller hospitals' management and physicians must consider as they explore opportunities for improvement. As patients begin to recognize the cost-saving (and life-saving!) advantages of early detection of illness and physicians realize the need to be more efficient care deliverers due to payment restrictions, the inherent qualities of a smaller local hospital will become more and more important.

Providing Education and Feedback

Ongoing education and feedback can have a significant effect on enhancing physician behavior. Physicians are often unaware of the economic factors in clinical decision making, and education and feedback can improve this awareness. Educational programs can be designed with the intention of improving physician behavior through increased clinical knowledge and an appreciation of the costs of hospital services. Usually these educational efforts have a short-term effect on reducing physician-generated costs. Education must be combined with repeated follow-up reinforcement to achieve any long-term positive results.

Individual cost-per-case weight-adjusted discharge information can be developed for and reported to each physician. A physician profile comparing individual physicians to their peer group can be very effective. The effect of this approach is improved significantly as the profiles are individualized to each physician's situation and new profiles are developed periodically.

Feedback to physicians on how their practice habits compare with ordering protocols, objective standards, and peer performance must take place if physicians are expected to change their behavior over the long term. Feedback reinforces a physician's sense of accomplishment and desire to provide excellent, cost-effective care along with his or her peers.

Overcoming Barriers to Collaboration

There are few things a hospital CEO values more than close, harmonious relationships with the members of the institution's medical staff. Utilization review has traditionally been a subject that has pitted CEOs against medical staff, eclipsing any other area of conflict. Often, utilization review dialogue between management and the medical staff only occurs when a physician has a patient in the hospital beyond the standard allotted length of stay. Historically, physicians and administrators have not been able to overcome the institutional barriers to cost containment.

Even though adequate incentives may be present, there are significant administrative and medical staff misgivings about utilization management that must be addressed before cost-containment initiatives can be successful. For administrators, programs designed to change physician practice behavior take management time, staff time, data-processing capacity, space, and other costly resources in a resource-limited facility (all hospitals are resource limited; smaller hospitals are just more limited than others). Some of the barriers to collaborative relationships facing physicians include conflicting medical staff opinions, insufficient scheduling and staffing models, a lack of meaningful information, and a shortage of alternative facilities.

Handling Variations in Medical Opinions

Variations in utilization rates are greater for cases in which physicians have more discretion in the choice of treatments. More variations in resource consumption are possible in treating uterine cancer than in treating a ruptured appendix. As discretion in treatment increases, the chance for standard treatment protocols is reduced.

Although some may argue this point, financial incentives can play a part in diagnosis and treatment decisions. In the past, physicians have continued to be paid for each hospital visit, even beyond the Medicare-allotted stay. Carriers are beginning to look at this policy and in some cases are reducing payment to physicians for excessive hospital visits.

Developing Efficient Scheduling

One of the most important things a hospital can offer a physician is enough flexibility to allow him or her to perform as many procedures as possible within a given amount of time. Efficient scheduling and adequate skilled labor support for patient care are critical in maintaining a positive medical staff relationship and utilization control. Unfortunately, hospitals have continued to look for ways to reduce payroll costs in light of payment cuts. If hospitals make payroll cuts without following a viable staffing model, resource consumption may increase instead of decrease and physician relations may be strained further.

Sharing Meaningful Information

Beyond monitoring length of stay and comparing charges to payments, a hospital often has very few meaningful data on which to base appropriate levels of utilization. Additionally, many hospitals have been reluctant to share extensive financial data with their physicians. More often than not, however, the sharing of information accelerates the collaborative progress. Physicians who understand the impact that they individually can have on the institution's viability are more likely to help develop and implement cost-containment measures.

Finding Alternative Facilities

Often, a physician is unable to discharge a patient to a skilled nursing home or another appropriate extended care setting because of the lack of available beds within what the patient or patient's family would consider an acceptable proximity to home. However, this attitude can change when financial incentives change. More and more hospitals are issuing termination-of-benefit (TOB) letters to guarantors of patients after their Medicare coverage expires. In these TOB letters, the guarantor is notified that the guarantor is responsible for paying the patient's bills. Upon receipt of such notice, a family may reconsider the issue of proximity.

Hospital–Physician Collaboration

Recognizing the barriers and challenges to reducing costs and improving outcomes, hospitals and physicians will have to creatively develop solutions. During the 1990s, cost-containment efforts will focus more on physician practice habits and how the treatment of patients is reported. Employers and other payers will demand more responsibility from all providers in controlling costs. This period will be particularly challenging for physicians accustomed to a high level of autonomy in the delivery of care. The more meaningful information the hospital can provide to its medical staff about the way patients are being treated, the better the opportunity will be for successful hospital–physician collaboration in making improvements.

Note

1. The relative case weights are assigned for each DRG by HCFA and updated on an annual basis. The case weights for all DRGs are published annually in the *Federal Register.* The case weights used in this example are for the year 1992.

Chapter 7

A Prelude to Managed Care

By 1995 nationwide, the combined enrollment of health maintenance organizations (HMOs) and preferred provider organizations (PPOs) will significantly dwarf the enrollment of traditional indemnity plans. This growth will result in contracting opportunities for hospitals and their medical staffs in PPOs. Most segments of the payer market (including Medicare) are now considering a shift to managed care systems. This shift will mean a dramatic change in the way health care is provided and paid for.

The primary goals of virtually all health care reform initiatives relate to three major areas: improved quality, increased access, and reduced costs. To meet these objectives, particularly cost containment, Medicare, Medicaid, commercial insurance carriers, and self-insured employers all continue to explore managed care alternatives. New payment and delivery systems that can expand access for their beneficiaries and reduce costs are the goal.

Under the current health care system, these seem like contradictory objectives. Hospitals are currently paid more for treating more acutely ill patients. There should be more incentives for maintaining health and preventing illness in order to keep more patients out of the hospital's acute care setting. Progress toward a better health care system can and must be made to meet the demands of the next decade and beyond. Progress will first require a change in basic attitudes and then comprehensive reform in the hospital payment system and the way smaller hospitals provide health care.

Trends in the Managed Care Market

The health care field is in the midst of a fundamental transition toward managed health care delivery systems as PPOs and HMOs experience unprecedented rates of growth at the expense of traditional indemnity insurance plans. Although this growth has been the fastest in urban areas, most experts recognize that economics will soon force employers nationwide to alter employee benefit plans, encouraging greater managed care enrollment. Employers in rural areas have been slower to embrace managed care, but this trend may very well change.

Helping to accelerate the transition to managed care has been the introduction of Medicare's Physician Payment Reform, the first major step by a third party to dissolve the traditional fee-for-service payment method. Most payment experts believe that other insurance companies will move to similar payment designs, and many believe that Medicare's Resource-Based Relative Value Scale (RBRVS) will be an effective way to contain costs. Other health care professionals are concerned that if a similar payment method is not adopted, physicians will attempt to shift higher charges to their insurance plans in order to offset losses from Medicare's payment reductions. As the result of a dwindling fee-for-service environment, managed care plans may soon seem both inevitable and acceptable to physicians.

Medicare is also experimenting with a managed care approach to health care cost reduction through its private health plan option. Through this plan, HMOs enter into a Medicare risk contract with the government. Under the Medicare risk contract, participating HMOs are paid 95 percent of what the federal government actuaries estimate to be the cost of services if the services were obtained under a fee-for-service arrangement.

This rapid growth in alternative delivery systems membership substantially strengthens the ability of PPOs and HMOs to control health care system trends as the organizations negotiate with a hospital field suffering from overcapacity. Hospitals and their medical staffs will certainly feel the impact of PPO and HMO growth. Although the precise future of the managed care market remains uncertain, several trends are emerging.

The Shift Away from the Sole Provider

Many health care experts argue that a smaller rural hospital is immune to the effects of managed care when it is the only hospital in the county. This sole provider status is thought by some administrators to eliminate hospital incentives to provide discounted or capitated rates to employers or managed care entities. The hospital and its medical staff will inevitably get all the patients from area employers and managed care entities, according to this reasoning. Even today, however, this is rarely the case.

Most smaller rural hospitals experience outmigration of insurance-paying patients because patients perceive larger hospitals to be better.

When patients are seriously ill, they require sophisticated specialists available only in urban areas or at large rural referral centers. To maintain or gain market share, smaller and rural hospitals must increase community awareness of services available through the hospital and its medical staff and make the hospital appear more inviting. The hospitals must also maintain a sufficient number of physicians on staff while continuing to be cost-attractive to those paying the bills. In addition, smaller and rural hospitals must demonstrate their ability to provide high-quality care and to provide or arrange for specialty care as needed. These are not easily attainable objectives.

The Arrival of Capitation

Capitation is often considered a four-letter word among health care providers. However, current health care reform may incorporate this structure of payment for hospital services. Under *capitation*, hospitals are reimbursed on a per-beneficiary per-month basis for all institutional costs for a defined population of beneficiaries. The amount of payment received may depend on the age and gender of the patient, but it does not vary with premium revenue. A derivative of capitated reimbursement pays hospitals a percentage of revenue from the premiums paid for beneficiaries to be enrolled in a plan. In both cases, a hospital is at risk for the costs of the services it performs. When a hospital is not capable of delivering certain levels of care, the cost for care that must be provided elsewhere is deducted from the capitation rate or percentage of revenue the hospital would otherwise receive.

The Transfer of Risk

In coming years, payers will continue to transfer risk from themselves to the health care providers serving their clientele. Payers will provide a patient referral base in exchange for this shared risk. The changing ways hospitals will provide services in this "managed" environment will be dramatic. As risk continues to shift, the cost of providing health care services will become more important than the number of patient days a hospital is experiencing.

In this new environment, revenue will no longer be based on the number of admissions, outpatient visits, or tests performed in ancillary departments. Instead, revenue will be based on a percentage of premiums paid by enrollees in each plan contracted by the provider. Hospitals, therefore, will be at risk for providing cost-effective health care to those enrollees. The less expensive a patient's treatment, the more profitable the provider will remain. Furthermore, hospitals and physicians will be evaluated and rewarded on the basis of clinical outcomes as well as costs.

Payers will place providers at risk to provide the best value in both containing costs and improving outcomes.

The Search for Market Share

The objectives of providers, payers, and beneficiaries are not always the same. In the coming managed care environment, the primary objective of employees and employers will be to receive the needed care at an acceptable level of quality and at the lowest cost. Hospitals and other providers will find themselves linked in the common objective of gaining or preserving market share. The measurement used by payers to award market share will be the degree of cost-effective delivery of care. Suddenly the critical questions of care will become how sick versus how much care and how many years of symptom-free living after care was delivered. Hospitals are not very comfortable with these questions because most hospitals do not have the answers.

The Proliferation of Health Plans

The managed care market will not be dominated by any one organization. Although national insurance companies and HMOs will capture a significant market share, local health plan organizations will also exist based on their ability to offer unique, custom-developed managed care products for specific communities and regions. What works in one region, and for one employer, may not work in another region for another employer.

The Dependency on Local Providers

Both national and local health plans will rely on the quality and efficiency of local delivery systems for their ultimate success. Providers who can demonstrate high quality and low cost profiles will have the best opportunity to contract with area health plans. Local hospitals and physicians may have opportunities to sponsor their own local health plans in some markets. Smaller hospitals will need to carefully select networks that can help them attain their strategic objectives. It will also be important for smaller hospitals to develop provider arrangements with local employers wherever possible.

The Measurability of Performance Standards

Payers will select high-quality providers with convenient locations and competitive prices. Large hospitals that have enjoyed a reputation for providing high-quality care because of their size will have new, measurable standards of performance to reach. As the expectations of customers change, smaller and rural hospitals will have a new, fairer playing field if they can meet these customer expectations. Utilization controls will be critical in maintaining competitive prices that will establish a hospital's market position.

The Collaboration of Providers

An integrated hospital–physician economic unit will be in the best position to negotiate with payers. Arriving at this position will require an open forum for identifying new methods to contain costs while delivering expected outcomes in the delivery of care. Hospitals will need to picture themselves as facilitators of care for their patients, their community, and all of their other "customers," including the ones who pay the bill. Managed care inherently changes the focus of health care delivery as hospitals manage patient care rather than departments and serve payers rather than physicians. Physicians will increasingly view themselves as a provider partner with the hospital.

Managed Care and Smaller Hospitals

In the coming managed care environment, smaller hospitals must become cost-effective and provide the bulk of health care services for their community. Three strategic elements will be required: provision of services that detect illness in its earliest stages; provision of such services efficiently as well as effectively; and involvement in a regional referral network of care. Some small hospitals may already be able to offer a wider array of services that go beyond primary care and diagnostic services. Others will have to develop networks of providers. Those hospitals that can manage the course of treatment for an entire population and establish contracting relationships with payers will be in the best strategic position.

Smaller hospitals with medical staffs that are accessible to plan enrollees for primary medicine will enjoy a distinct advantage. Smaller hospitals can be the access point to a provider network and can solidify its market position by establishing contractual relationships with local employers, physicians, and regional referral centers. The ability to manage cases will become as important as the ability to perform a heart transplant. Employers will seek those providers who can demonstrate the ability to conform to their plan requirements in providing the health care management function.

In the future, it appears that all hospitals either will be part of a managed care network or will administer their own managed care plans with the assistance of other providers that will contract with the hospital's network. As a result, hospitals must understand some common methods used to contain costs in managed care organizations.

Preadmission Testing and Same-Day Surgery

One of the simplest and most common cost-control methods used by managed care organizations is preadmission testing and same-day surgery for procedures performed on an elective basis. Under this arrangement, members of a managed care plan undergo routine preoperative testing as outpatients. Test results are sent to the admitting physician, who performs the history and physical in his or her office or at the hospital on an outpatient basis. The physician delivers, sends, or calls in the results of the history and physical to the hospital, including all test results. The patient is then admitted to the hospital's same-day surgery department the day of the surgery and may be discharged after a short recovery period depending on the patient's condition. Same-day surgery does not, however, explicitly require outpatient surgery.

Often, a managed care plan may make arrangements with an outside laboratory to provide the preadmission testing at a rate significantly below a hospital's established price. In this case, the hospital may be forced to match this lower price if it wants to capture this part of the business. If the outside lab is accredited and can demonstrate accurate and timely reporting of results, its use would appear to be a cost-effective alternative to hospital testing. The hospital will need to accept outside lab reports or expect to see elective surgery referrals sent to a more cooperative hospital.

Mandatory Outpatient Surgery

Many managed care plans have designated a list of surgical procedures that may only be performed on an outpatient basis unless prior approval is obtained from the plan's medical director. Unfortunately, no two managed care plans are identical, making the precertification process very difficult for hospitals. To avoid the confusion, it is probably wise for hospitals to steer all medically appropriate patients to the ambulatory setting for surgery. The managed care entity must be careful when using the mandatory outpatient surgery rule. Charges associated with the outpatient procedure can at times exceed the amount the plan would have paid if the patient had been admitted as an inpatient.

Maximum Allowable Length of Stay

Assigning a maximum allowable length of stay (MaxLOS) is also a common method of cost control used by managed care organizations. In a similar fashion to the Medicare DRG system, the MaxLOS is determined by the diagnosis and the ICD-9-CM code assignment. Managed care plans assign a MaxLOS based on the principal admission diagnosis. If a patient is admitted for appendicitis and an appendectomy is performed, the patient may be awarded a four-day stay as the MaxLOS. If the patient stays six days, payment will be received for only the allowed four days.

Key Roles in Medical Management

In an environment requiring increased emphasis on managing the cost of treatment, the roles of precertification, utilization review, and discharge planning will become more and more important. These functions depend on the skill of the managed care entity's utilization review coordinator, primary care physician, and consulting physician.

The Utilization Review Coordinator

Utilization review is critical to the success of managed care programs. This function serves as the eyes and ears of medical management. The responsibilities of utilization managers vary based on the expectations of a given plan. Usually, the clinical nature of the information required for utilization management calls for the coordinator to be the utilization reviewer. The more common responsibilities of a utilization review coordinator are described in the following paragraphs.

Information Gathering

Accurate information concerning hospital cases must be obtained in a timely fashion. Necessary case information includes:

- The admission date and diagnosis
- The service area of the hospital (medical, surgical, obstetrics, and so forth)
- The physicians involved in the patient's case (who is the admitting physician, consulting physician, and so forth)
- The planned procedures
- The expected discharge date
- The specific needs related to discharge planning

Typically, the utilization reviewers ensure that this information is obtained and distributed to other members of the medical management team and claims department personnel.

Case information is gathered primarily through the use of telephone and hospital rounding. Telephone rounding is used when extensive geographic coverage requirements restrict the utilization review coordinator's ability to gather information in person. For other care plans where providers are in closer geographic proximity and labor resources are greater, the utilization review coordinator can visit every hospitalized member of the plan. The conflict between these two rounding alternatives is the quality and detail of case information versus the expense entailed in obtaining the information.

Discharge Planning

Discharge planning begins at the time or before a patient is admitted. Effective discharge planning requires the physician and the utilization review coordinator to consider this function to be part of the patient's overall treatment plan. As hospitals become more skilled at developing patient protocols, they will also improve in the discharge planning function. Discharge planning includes an estimate of the patient's length of stay, the patient's expected outcome, special patient requirements upon discharge, as well as a prioritization of patient concerns to be facilitated.

For example, suppose a patient is diagnosed to have a fractured hip. It is identified early that the patient will need several weeks of rehabilitation, and so a rehabilitation facility is immediately contacted and given an expected day of discharge from the hospital so that the facility can reserve a bed for the patient. If it is evident that the patient will need durable medical equipment (DME), the equipment should also be ordered at this time. If the patient is placed on a waiting list for the rehabilitation bed or if the DME provider must order the needed equipment for the patient, then some or all of the waiting period can be absorbed during the patient's length of stay in the hospital. Early discharge planning is obviously in the best interest of the patient as well as the hospital's cost-containment objectives.

Often overlooked is the importance of informing patients and their families of discharge planning issues. If patients are not periodically updated, they may be somewhat surprised when their physicians announce that they are going to be discharged. If patients and their families are not prepared for discharge to home or to another facility, physicians may be inclined to extend hospital stays. Unfortunately, the costs and iatrogenic risks associated with an additional hospital day are unacceptably high for patients who are healthy enough to be discharged.

In a smaller hospital, the utilization review coordinator is in the best position to coordinate the discharge planning effort. In addition to ensuring a timely and appropriate discharge, the utilization review coordinator can also follow up with the patient after discharge to make sure the patient is doing well.

The Primary Care Physician

In the managed care environment, it is the primary care physician's role to make daily rounds and coordinate patient care. When a patient is receiving care from a consulting physician, it is even more important that a primary care physician makes daily rounds. Daily rounds help ensure that continuity of care is delivered while the patient is in the hospital, and they provide a comforting presence to the patient. As a result, the patient develops a closer relationship with the primary care physician, which is a critical element in the health care continuum.

By monitoring a patient's clinical course of treatment and discharge plan, the primary care physician will be in a better position to manage the patient's case after discharge. And this effective patient management enables the primary care physician to have a major effect on proper utilization of health care resources.

As more physicians become involved with a patient, the harder it becomes to control the cost and quality of care being rendered. Often, a patient's primary care physician feels uncomfortable in confronting actions taken by the consulting physicians. To reduce this lack of comfort, primary care physicians should try the following suggestions when working with consulting physicians:

- Discuss the case with the consultant and suggest methods to reduce resource consumption and length of stay.
- Communicate with the consulting physician in the event that the consulting physician failed to make rounds. For example, in a surgery case, the primary care physician might be able to communicate to the surgeon that a patient appears to be ready for discharge when the surgeon has not yet seen the patient that day. After discussing the patient's condition with the surgeon, the primary care physician could arrange the discharge.

In the managed care environment, the primary care physician is responsible for the medical management of the patient. This responsibility includes determining a reasonably expected outcome as well as the financial soundness of providing prescribed care. As a result, the primary care physician must consider new ways of caring for patients that ensure high quality and cost-effectiveness. Primary care physicians must remember that they are responsible for their patients' care and that the consulting physician is just a consultant. The primary care physician has every right to ask questions related to the way a consultant is treating a case. A better understanding of physician roles by all parties results in greater opportunity to control resource utilization.

The Consulting Physician

Although most managed care plans emphasize the primary care physician's role, consulting specialists are usually the most resource-consumptive physicians. A managed care entity has some basic expectations regarding patient management by the consulting physician, including:

- Being aware of the managed care plan's policy on testing, procedures, and primary care case management
- Keeping the primary care physician aware of the status of the patient
- Directing patient care back to the primary care physician as soon as the care level is deemed appropriate
- Authorizing further patient care only after discussion with the primary care physician

If these guidelines are followed, resource consumption by consulting physicians can be reduced.

Credentialing in Open and Closed Panels

The credentialing process in any setting is more than a verification of the physician's licensure. Credentialing involves the delineation of physician privileges that specify what each physician is permitted to do based on demonstrated clinical competence, education, and training. Physician involvement in managed care plans is controlled by two types of credentialing panels. In a closed panel plan, the managed care entity contracts with a limited number of physicians. Members of a plan that uses a closed panel are not allowed to visit physicians who are not part of this exclusive, limited group of physicians. If the managed care entity utilizes an open panel, then participation in the managed care plan will be open to any physician who meets the plan's credentialing criteria.

Credentialing new physicians in closed panels is quite different from credentialing in open panels. *Credentialing* entails ensuring that the physicians who apply have the necessary documents as evidence of sufficient medical competence to practice within a managed care plan. In open panels, the physician is responsible for obtaining the necessary documentation. In closed panels, it is the plan's responsibility to obtain this information for the physician.

Selecting physicians for the credentialing panels is a critical process in maintaining quality and cost control. Careful control and analysis in the selection of physicians and other providers may permit the managed care entity to concentrate its recruiting efforts on qualified and reputable providers. There will still, however, be a few member physicians who are not able to meet panel standards. Because managed care entities are expected to create an environment that encourages efficient health care delivery in a competitive marketplace, physicians unable to conform to the plan's expectations should not be permitted to participate.

Controlling Ancillary Costs

Although much emphasis has traditionally been placed on controlling length of patient stay, managed care organizations have found that ancillary and emergency services consume a growing portion of plan resources. It is difficult to control ancillary expenses through financial incentives for plan members because patients rarely seek these services without a physician referral. Even if a patient did self-refer for ancillary or emergency services, it is unlikely that a health care facility would administer the care without a referral from a physician.

Control of these services depends on the utilization patterns of the referring physicians. Monitoring physician patterns and identifying ways to be more cost-effective is as valuable to the physician as it is to the hospital. The managed care entity may very well establish standards of care for the physician to follow. If the managed care entity has not developed such standards, other alternatives might include continual tests of reasonableness, limits on the number of visits for treatment without prior approval, and limits on the authority to order ancillary services.

Continual tests of reasonableness are usually utilized if standards of care have not been developed by a managed care entity. In this approach, the managed care entity continually reviews the tests being ordered by the referring physician to evaluate whether the information being collected will have an effect on the care being delivered. For example, a review may indicate that patients receive a chest X ray as part of a physician's normal admitting routine, even when the test is unrelated to the admitting diagnosis. If a patient's condition fails to show any improvement over an extended period of time, continuation of prescribed therapy may also be questioned.

Managed care entities may also limit the number of times a therapy may be delivered. For example, a provider may be limited to administering only three or four physical therapy treatments. If the provider wishes to administer additional treatments, the physical therapist and primary care physician would need to submit a specific care plan for approval. In other cases, a treatment plan is developed upon patient admission, with approval for the number of tests secured early in the patient's stay based on the initial plan.

Some managed care plans may also attempt to control the use of ancillary services by limiting the physicians' authority to order tests. This method is usually more common among HMOs. Although often impractical, some plans call for a consulting physician to discuss the ordering of any patient tests with the patient's primary care physician, and it is the primary care physician who must order the tests.

Managed care organizations have as much incentive to prospectively control the use of ancillaries as do providers. Providers run the risk of administering more care than the plan will financially accommodate. The managed care plan's incentive is to avoid paying the maximum limit for tests with each case.

Being Postured for Change

It is hard to devote a great deal of attention to the managed care environment when it does not represent a significant portion of the hospital's market share. The managed care environment as it is today, however, has many characteristics of the emerging health care market. To survive, hospitals must be able to continue operating under the current rules of health care delivery and payment and have an organization and approach in place for the forthcoming environment.

The new health care environment will call for hospitals to do some things in new ways. It will also ask hospitals to do the things that successful hospitals have been doing for a long time. (There's truth in the adage "the more things change, the more things stay the same.") Hospitals must continue to foster a creative environment in improving the hospital processes while maintaining close control over staffing, supply costs, and inventory. Hospitals will need to work more closely with physicians in delivering the most efficient care possible. Budgets must be used in planning and evaluating departmental as well as hospital performance.

Perhaps most important, an environment must be created and nurtured that will allow for the attainment of hospital objectives through the voluntary actions and cooperation of physicians, employees, managers, and trustees. Better quality and access to care can only happen when everyone does their part.

Additional Books of Interest

Investment Program Management for Health Care Institutions

by Gregory C. Krohm, Ph.D., Mary P. Merrill, M.B.A., C.F.P., and Alan B. Talarczyk, J.D., C.P.A.

". . . [an] excellent book . . . should be useful to graduate students and health-care financial managers unfamiliar with investment program management."

> Steven R. Eastaugh, ScD, professor of finance and health economics, George Washington University, Washington, DC in *Healthcare Financial Management*

An easy-to-follow nontechnical text, this book assists administrators, chief financial officers, and trustees to make more informed investment management decisions. It provides clear instructions on writing an investment program policy statement and contains guidelines for choosing, managing, and evaluating the performance of investment managers. The authors help you understand your investment needs, explain the basic investment terms and concepts, and help you make sense of the macroeconomy.

1991. 145 pages, 11 figures, 7 tables.
ISBN 1-55648-058-X Catalog No. E99-061153
$44.95 (AHA members, $35.95)

Engineering a Hospital Turnaround: Proven Strategies for Reinvigorating Financial and Operating Performance

edited by Richard A. Baehr for Ernst & Young

Methodologies for recognizing the warning signals of hospital distress and for gaining financial and operational health to ensure long-term viability. The twenty contributors discuss: revenue and cash enhancement, market and program repositioning, medical staff issues, cost reduction and quality improvement, capital restructuring, phaseout options, and bankruptcies versus workouts. Case studies profile the turnaround of a multihospital system and an independent community hospital.

1993. 228 pages.
ISBN 1-55648-102-0 Catalog No. E99-001120
$45.00 (AHA members, $36.00)

To order, call TOLL FREE
1-800-AHA-2626